Iron Deficiency Anemia:
Recommended Guidelines for the Prevention, Detection, and Management Among U.S. Children and Women of Childbearing Age

Committee on the Prevention, Detection, and
Management of Iron Deficiency Anemia Among
U.S. Children and Women of Childbearing Age

FOOD AND NUTRITION BOARD
INSTITUTE OF MEDICINE

Robert Earl and Catherine E. Woteki, Editors

National Academy Press
Washington, D.C. 1993

National Academy Press • 2101 Constitution Avenue, N.W. • Washington, D.C. 20418

NOTICE: The project that is the subject of this report was approved by the Governing Board of the National Research Council, whose members are drawn from the councils of the National Academy of Sciences, the National Academy of Engineering, and the Institute of Medicine. The members of the committee responsible for the report were chosen for their special competences and with regard for appropriate balance.

This report has been reviewed by a group other than the authors according to procedures approved by a Report Review Committee consisting of members of the National Academy of Sciences, the National Academy of Engineering, and the Institute of Medicine.

The Institute of Medicine was chartered in 1970 by the National Academy of Sciences to enlist distinguished members of the appropriate professions in the examination of policy matters pertaining to the health of the public. In this, the Institute acts under both the Academy's 1863 congressional charter responsibility to be an adviser to the federal government and its own initiative in identifying issues of medical care, research, and education. Dr. Kenneth I. Shine is president of the Institute of Medicine.

This study was supported under contract no. 200-92-0574 from the Division of Nutrition, Centers for Disease Control and Prevention, Public Health Service, U.S. Department of Health and Human Services.

Library of Congress Catalog Card No. 93-86771

International Standard Book Number 0-309-04987-3

Additional copies of this report are available from:

National Academy Press
2101 Constitution Avenue, N.W.
Box 285
Washington, DC 20055

Call 800-624-6242 or 202-334-3313 (in the Washington metropolitan area).

B245

Copyright 1993 by the National Academy of Sciences. All rights reserved.

Printed in the United States of America

The serpent has been a symbol of long life, healing, and knowledge among almost all cultures and religions since the beginning of recorded history. The image adopted as a logotype by the Institute of Medicine is based on a relief carving from ancient Greece, now held by the Staatlichemuseen in Berlin.

COMMITTEE ON THE PREVENTION, DETECTION, AND MANAGEMENT OF IRON DEFICIENCY ANEMIA AMONG U.S. CHILDREN AND WOMEN OF CHILDBEARING AGE

DORIS H. CALLOWAY (*Chair*),* Department of Nutrition, University of California, Berkeley, California

JOHN L. BEARD, Nutrition Department and Department of Biobehavioral Health, College of Health and Human Development, The Pennsylvania State University, University Park, Pennsylvania

JAMES D. COOK, Division of Hematology, University of Kansas Medical Center, Kansas City, Kansas

SAMUEL J. FOMON, Department of Pediatrics, University of Iowa Hospitals, Iowa City, Iowa

JANET L. MITCHELL, Department of Obstetrics and Gynecology, Harlem Hospital Center, New York, New York

DAVID RUSH, Epidemiology Program, USDA Human Nutrition Research Center on Aging at Tufts University, Boston, Massachusetts

Consultants

GEORGE H. BEATON, Department of Nutrition Science, University of Toronto, Toronto, Ontario, Canada

PETER R. DALLMAN, Contract Writer, San Francisco, California

* Member, Institute of Medicine

Staff

CATHERINE E. WOTEKI, Project Director
ROBERT EARL, Program Officer
MARCIA S. LEWIS, Project Assistant
MICHAEL K. HAYES, Editorial Consultant

FOOD AND NUTRITION BOARD

M.R.C. GREENWOOD (*Chair*),* Office of Graduate Studies, University of California, Davis, California
EDWIN L. BIERMAN (*Vice Chair*),* Division of Metabolism, Endocrinology, and Nutrition, University of Washington, Seattle, Washington
PERRY L. ADKISSON,† Department of Entomology, Texas A&M University, College Station, Texas
LINDSAY ALLEN, Department of Nutrition, University of California, Davis, California
DENNIS M. BIER, Pediatric Clinical Research Center, Washington University School of Medicine, St. Louis, Missouri
HECTOR F. DeLUCA,† Department of Biochemistry, University of Wisconsin, Madison, Wisconsin
MICHAEL P. DOYLE, Department of Food Science and Technology, Georgia Experiment Station, University of Georgia, Griffin, Georgia
JOHANNA T. DWYER, Frances Stern Nutrition Center, New England Medical Center Hospital, Boston, Massachusetts
JOHN W. ERDMAN, JR., Department of Food Science and Division of Nutritional Sciences, College of Agriculture, University of Illinois, Urbana, Illinois
CUTBERTO GARZA, Division of Nutritional Sciences, Cornell University, Ithaca, New York
K. MICHAEL HAMBIDGE, Department of Pediatrics, University of Colorado Medical Center, Denver, Colorado
JANET C. KING, Department of Nutritional Sciences, University of California, Berkeley, California
JOHN E. KINSELLA (*deceased*), School of Agriculture and Environmental Sciences, University of California, Davis, California
LAURENCE N. KOLONEL, Cancer Center of Hawaii, University of Hawaii, Honolulu, Hawaii
SANFORD A. MILLER, Graduate Studies and Biological Sciences, University of Texas Health Science Center, San Antonio, Texas
ARTHUR H. RUBENSTEIN (*IOM Council Liaison*),* Department of Medicine, The University of Chicago, Chicago, Illinois
ALFRED SOMMER,* School of Hygiene and Public Health, Johns Hopkins University, Baltimore, Maryland
STEVE L. TAYLOR (*ex officio*), Department of Food Science and Technology, University of Nebraska, Lincoln, Nebraska
VERNON R. YOUNG,† School of Science, Massachusetts Institute of Technology, Cambridge, Massachusetts

* Member, Institute of Medicine
† Member, National Academy of Sciences

Staff

CATHERINE E. WOTEKI, Director
MARCIA S. LEWIS, Administrative Assistant
SUSAN M. WYATT, Financial Associate

Preface

Over the last decade, several expert groups have addressed the issue of iron deficiency anemia in young children and women of childbearing age. Dietary allowances have been revised, diagnostic criteria for defining anemia have been promulgated, and preventive and therapeutic measures have been developed and, for the most part, implemented. So, why another examination of the issue?

There are several reasons why a responsible agency would undertake such a reexamination. There are seemingly straightforward questions about the continued necessity for and effectiveness of existing programs. These questions are, however, complex and difficult to answer because the information base is not entirely secure. The answers to such problematic questions depend on a reasoned judgment as to the significance of new epidemiologic evidence and other scientific findings and on an ability to forecast trends. In the present instance account needs to be taken of, inter alia, trends in the consumption and composition of foods and changes in the nutritional environment more generally.

It is to be expected that committee members will not always be in perfect accord in the absence of sufficient, solid information. Members' judgments are influenced by their different experiences and disciplinary backgrounds. The present committee resolved this problem by accepting an argument that in order to set aside the recommendations of other expert groups, the contravening evidence must be as strong as the evidence that led to the others' decisions. The guidelines developed by the present committee are substantially in accord with existing recommendations. The committee did note areas of uncertainty and urges that high priority be given to developing the information needed to improve decision making. Some points are noted in the text, and an indicative list of research topics is included in the report.

The committee's work was assisted very greatly by the background documentation prepared by Dr. Peter Dallman in a consultative capacity; we acknowledge his major contribution and appreciate the willingness with which he undertook revision as issues arose. Dr. Dallman participated in all deliberations of the committee as a member de facto. Professor George Beaton was available for consultation only at our last meeting; his ability to pose important clarifying questions was, as always, greatly appreciated. The committee owes a special debt to two of its members—to Professor John L. Beard for providing background on iron-dependent pathologies and to Dr. David Rush for a new analysis of data from the U.S. Department of Agriculture's Special Supplemental Food Program for Women, Infants, and Children and for solicitation of additional views and references relating to iron supplementation during pregnancy.

We wish particularly to thank Dr. Anne Looker and Dr. Christopher Sempos and their colleagues at the National Center for Health Statistics who prepared preliminary analyses of data from the third National Health and Nutrition Examination Survey and shared other, as yet unpublished, work.

I wish personally to thank the committee members for their diligence and patience, and for the care and concern they showed for those whom the guidelines are intended to benefit. None of the committee's tasks could have been accomplished without the leadership of Dr. Catherine Woteki and the support of her staff, especially Mr. Robert Earl and Ms. Marcia Lewis. We are grateful for their unfailing courtesy and generosity and commend the high standards reflected in their professional contributions.

DORIS HOWES CALLOWAY, *Chair*
Committee on the Prevention, Detection,
and Management of Iron Deficiency
Anemia Among U.S. Children and
Women of Childbearing Age

Contents

THE COMMITTEE'S CHARGE AND APPROACH 1

MAJOR ISSUES 2
    Defining Anemia, 3
    Prevalence of Anemia as a Public Health Problem, 5
    Implications of Research on Excess Iron Intake, 7
    Developing Screening and Intervention Guidelines, 8
    Intervention Strategies: Efficacy and Safety, 9
    Supplementation for Infants and Children, 10
    Supplementation for Women, 10
    Safety, 11

RECOMMENDED GUIDELINES FOR PREVENTION, DETECTION, AND MANAGEMENT OF IRON DEFICIENCY ANEMIA 11
    Infants and Children, 14
    Nonpregnant Women of Childbearing Age, 15
    Pregnant Women, 16
    Comments and Caution About Cutoff Values for Laboratory Tests, 18
    Comments and Caution About Routine Use of Ferritin Values, 18

RECOMMENDED GUIDELINES FOR PREVENTING AND TREATING IRON DEFICIENCY ANEMIA IN INFANTS AND CHILDREN 20

RECOMMENDED GUIDELINES FOR PREVENTING AND TREATING IRON DEFICIENCY ANEMIA IN NONPREGNANT WOMEN OF CHILDBEARING AGE 22

RECOMMENDED GUIDELINES FOR PREVENTING AND TREATING IRON DEFICIENCY ANEMIA IN PREGNANT WOMEN 24

RECOMMENDATIONS FOR RESEARCH 26
Efficacy of Routine Iron Supplementation During Pregnancy, 26
Research Base for Public Policy, 29

REFERENCES 32

APPENDIXES

A Acknowledgments, 39

B Iron Deficiency Anemia: A Synthesis of Current Scientific Knowledge and U.S. Recommendations for Prevention and Treatment,
Peter R. Dallman, 41

C Iron-Dependent Pathologies,
John L. Beard, 99

D Dietary Iron: Trends in the Iron Content of Foods, Use of Supplemental Iron, and the Framework for Regulation of Iron in the Diet, 113

E Committee and Staff Biographies, 123

Iron Deficiency Anemia:
Recommended Guidelines for the Prevention, Detection, and Management Among U.S. Children and Women of Childbearing Age

At the request of the Division of Nutrition, Centers for Disease Control and Prevention (CDC), Public Health Service, U.S. Department of Health and Human Services, the Committee on the Prevention, Detection, and Management of Iron Deficiency Anemia Among U.S. Children and Women of Childbearing Age was established under the auspices of the Food and Nutrition Board (FNB) of the Institute of Medicine (IOM) to prepare a report on the prevention, detection, and management of iron deficiency anemia in infants and young children and in women of childbearing age.

THE COMMITTEE'S CHARGE AND APPROACH

The committee's charge included the following:

1. to conduct a critical review of the information related to public health-oriented prevention, detection, and management of iron deficiency anemia, with primary emphasis on infants and children and secondary emphasis on women of childbearing age;
2. to develop specific guidelines and recommendations for the prevention, detection, and management of iron deficiency anemia in primary health care and public health clinic settings for both of these population groups, including ways to influence the roles of health care providers in these activities; and
3. to develop priorities for research related to a public health-oriented approach to the prevention, detection, and management of iron deficiency anemia.

The committee also was charged with considering the need for adaptations of the recommended guidelines, if any, for members of minority groups.

The six FNB committee members were selected for their expertise in iron nutrition, hematology, pediatrics, obstetrics and gynecology, and epidemiology. Because of the short time span of this project, the FNB commissioned a background paper in advance of the committee's first meeting. That paper—a comprehensive review of the science and current policy related to iron deficiency anemia—appears as Appendix B to this report. The committee met twice to read the background paper, collect and consider additional information, identify gaps in knowledge, and prepare draft guidelines as requested by the

CDC, and it met with representatives of federal agencies to determine how such guidelines might affect these agencies' activities.

This committee report summarizes information related to public health measures for the prevention, detection, and management of iron deficiency anemia, presents recommended guidelines related to this area as they apply in primary health care and public health clinic settings, and makes recommendations for research. The report identifies and addresses aspects that differ between the two target populations (infants and children, and women of childbearing age), as well as those common to both groups, and briefly considers family-oriented approaches. This report is intended to provide a frame of reference for health professionals and to assist the CDC with preparing national guidelines for the prevention and control of iron deficiency anemia. A fuller exposition of the information that informed the committee's deliberations is found in the appendixes to this report and in the references.

MAJOR ISSUES

In approaching its task, the committee considered several issues: the importance of iron deficiency anemia as a public health problem on the basis of prevalence estimates and health effects, the availabilities and efficacies of different public health approaches for prevention and detection, and the positive and negative implications of alternative approaches for the population at risk and the general population.

Two approaches can be taken to address public health problems: a population-based approach and an individual-based approach. When applied to reducing the prevalence of iron deficiency anemia, the population-based approach seeks to lower the population's risk by enriching and fortifying the food supply and by altering individual food choices through education and information programs. The individual-based approach seeks to identify those at the highest risk and to treat them by providing both supplements and education to increase the iron contents of their diets. The two approaches are complementary means of achieving lower rates of iron deficiency anemia.

After considering the alternative public health approaches and their consequences, the committee concluded that one major assumption had to be made before guidelines could be formulated: Iron enrichment and fortification of the U.S. food supply shall remain at current levels. In view of concerns about the adverse health effects attributable to the consumption of large amounts of iron, the committee believes that increasing the amount of fortification or the range of fortified products for the general population is not an appropriate public health strategy for preventing iron deficiency anemia (however, it may prove desirable to consider iron fortification of other foods specifically targeted at certain subgroups [e.g., infants]). Nor does the committee believe that currently available data allow it to recommend that the amount of fortification be lowered at this time. This situation may change as the nutrition and public health communities better understand the implication of the results of serum ferritin levels from the third National Health and Nutrition Examination Survey (NHANES III).

These conclusions were made on the basis of two observations. First, the prevalence of iron deficiency anemia among young children has been declining, and the decline is attributed to the use of iron-fortified formula and cereal, appropriate supplementation of breastfed infants, and later introduction of cow's milk to infants' diets than had been typical in the past. Second, preliminary data from the most recent national survey (NHANES III) indicate that average levels of serum ferritin, a marker of iron stores, have increased among adult males. If more detailed analyses confirm this observation, higher levels of iron enrichment and fortification of the general food supply would not be warranted because of the potential harm to those at risk of developing hemochromatosis.

The committee then considered the second available approach—that of screening individuals at risk to identify and treat those affected. This individual-based approach is appropriate because of the availability of tests with acceptable sensitivities and specificities, the prospect of the more widespread availability of new tests that detect iron depletion before the development of symptoms, and the availability of inexpensive iron supplements. The database supporting the beneficial effects of treating iron deficiency anemia in childhood is substantial, but the committee questioned the adequacy of the database demonstrating benefits from routine iron supplementation during pregnancy. This last issue is discussed more fully in the committee's recommendations for research.

Subsequent sections of the report discuss four major issues that the committee considered:

- defining iron deficiency anemia and the effects of different criteria on its estimated prevalence,
- determining the prevalence of iron deficiency anemia and considering its public health importance,
- developing methods for delivering iron to children and women, and
- determining the efficacy and safety of different interventions.

These issues and the committee's conclusions follow.

Defining Anemia

Anemia is defined as a hemoglobin concentration (or hematocrit) that is below the 95 percent confidence interval (i.e., below the 2.5th percentile) for healthy, well-nourished individuals of the same age, sex, and stage of pregnancy (LSRO, 1984). The cutoff values are from the population surveyed in NHANES II after exclusion of individuals with a high probability of iron deficiency (Table 1).

TABLE 1 Cutoff Values for Iron Deficiency Anemia in Children, Women of Childbearing Age, and Pregnant Women [a]

Group and Age (yr)	Hemoglobin Concentration (g/dl)	Hematocrit (%)
Children (both sexes)		
0.5–4.9	11.0	33
5.0–11.9	11.5	35
Women (≥12 yr)		
Nonpregnant	12.0	36
Pregnant, first trimester	11.0	33
Pregnant, second trimester	10.5	32
Pregnant, third trimester	11.5	34

[a] Hemoglobin values are rounded off to the nearest 0.5 g/dl, and hematocrit is rounded off to the nearest percent.

SOURCES: AAP, CON (1993); CDC (1989).

Iron deficiency anemia refers to an anemia that is associated with additional laboratory evidence of iron depletion as a result of one or more of the following tests results: low serum ferritin concentration, low transferrin saturation, or an elevation in the erythrocyte protoporphyrin level.

Iron deficiency without anemia represents a relatively mild iron deficiency that is diagnosed on the basis of a combination of biochemical indicators of iron status but in which the hemoglobin concentration remains within the normal range. Although no single indicator of iron status is diagnostic of functional iron deficiency, a low serum ferritin concentration indicates that iron reserves are depleted.

Hematologic Indicators of Iron Nutrition

Measurement of hemoglobin and hematocrit levels is used to screen for anemia and putative iron deficiency because they are easy and inexpensive to measure and reflect the largest iron compartment in the body. However, individuals with mild degrees of iron deficiency are missed by such screenings because of the overlap in values between normal and iron-deficient individuals. Hemoglobin and hematocrit values vary by age, sex, and stage of pregnancy. Hemoglobin values normally are lower in children than in nonpregnant adults. During puberty, the average hemoglobin concentration of males rises above that of females—a gender difference sustained throughout the reproductive years. During pregnancy, hemoglobin values gradually fall to a low point in the second trimester, largely because of a normal expansion in blood volume. From the end of the second trimester to term, the concentration of hemoglobin rises again. The average hemoglobin concentration of healthy blacks is lower than that of other races, by about 0.3 g/dl in young children and 0.8 g/dl in adults, as recorded in the NHANES II database.

Determination of the serum ferritin concentration is the only commonly used laboratory test that allows the evaluation of iron reserves. A serum ferritin concentration of less than 10 µg/liter in infants and children and less than 12 µg/liter in adults by itself indicates depleted iron stores. In combination with low hemoglobin or hematocrit levels, a serum ferritin concentration of less than 15 µg/liter in infants and children or less than 20 µg/liter in adults indicates iron deficiency anemia (LSRO, 1984). The serum ferritin concentration is elevated in the presence of infection and should be measured when the person is free of infectious disease (i.e., for at least 2 weeks).

Erythrocyte protoporphyrin accumulates in red blood cells when insufficient iron is available to form heme, the iron-containing portion of hemoglobin. Erythrocyte protoporphyrin levels are elevated in individuals with iron deficiency anemia or lead poisoning, as well as in those with infections or inflammatory conditions of more than 1 week in duration. In an otherwise healthy individual, anemia accompanied by an elevated protoporphyrin level is most commonly indicative of iron deficiency anemia.

Other laboratory tests used for the diagnosis of iron deficiency anemia include mean corpuscular volume (MCV), serum iron concentration and iron-binding capacity, and transferrin receptor concentration. A low MCV is most commonly associated with iron deficiency anemia or thalassemia trait; a high MCV but low hemoglobin is inconsistent with a diagnosis of iron deficiency and is more likely anemia caused by folate or vitamin B_{12} deficiency.

The ratio of serum iron to iron-binding capacity (transferrin saturation) is decreased in individuals with iron deficiency. This measure is less frequently used than in the past because the samples used for measurements can be easily contaminated and its reproducibility is relatively poor.

Transferrin receptor concentration is a promising new indicator that should shortly become available for widespread use. The transferrin receptor concentration is elevated in individuals with iron deficiency anemia but not in those with inflammatory disease, a useful feature (Ferguson et al., 1992). For nutritional survey purposes, the combination of transferrin receptor, serum ferritin, and hemoglobin concentration determinations is likely to provide an excellent depiction of iron status (Cook et al., 1993).

Prevalence of Anemia as a Public Health Problem

Current information on the prevalence of iron deficiency anemia in the United States comes from data collected between 1976 and 1980 as part of NHANES II. In NHANES II, the prevalence of iron deficiency anemia (determined by MCV, transferrin saturation, and erythrocyte protoporphyrin) was about 9 percent (those below the 95 percent confidence interval; i.e., below the 2.5th percentile) in children 12 to 24 months of age (LSRO, 1984). For nonpregnant women of childbearing age, the prevalence of iron deficiency anemia found in NHANES II was 5 percent. Throughout the 1980s, the prevalence of iron deficiency anemia in infants and preschool-age children declined, on the basis of prevalence data collected under the CDC Pediatric Surveillance System, from 7 to 3 percent (Yip et al., 1987a,b). Preliminary data from NHANES III collected between 1988 and 1991 appear to confirm this trend (preliminary analysis of data on hemoglobin and serum ferritin concentration measures only), with a prevalence at or below 3 percent for both black and white children 1 to 5 years of age; the prevalence among Mexican American infants, but not young children, may be somewhat higher (A.C. Looker, National Center for Health Statistics, personal communication, June 1993).

For women of childbearing age, data do not show a similar drop in the prevalence of iron deficiency anemia. NHANES II and preliminary NHANES III data show that 4 to 10 percent of U.S. women of childbearing age have iron deficiency anemia on the basis of two or three abnormal values for the surveyed indicators of iron status (see above). The estimated prevalence is lower in non-Hispanic white women than in black women and women in one Hispanic subgroup. Women between 15 and 19 years of age have a prevalence of iron deficiency anemia similar to that of women between 20 and 44 years of age. For women between 20 and 44 years of age, a higher prevalence of iron deficiency anemia is associated with poverty, low educational attainment, and high parity (LSRO, 1984).

No national population survey data on iron deficiency anemia are available for pregnant women. However, data on low-income women are available from the CDC Pregnancy Nutrition Surveillance System, and the national WIC evaluation. The 1990 CDC survey reported prevalences of iron deficiency anemia of 10, 14, and 33 percent in the first, second, and third trimesters of pregnancy, respectively, for all pregnant women of all races (Kim et al., 1992). Black women exhibited a significantly higher prevalence of iron deficiency anemia than did women of other races. CDC data show that the prevalence of iron deficiency anemia in the low-income population has remained stable since 1979, a finding that the committee found particularly troubling.

Data from the 1985 National WIC Evaluation were consistent with most past studies—a significant negative relationship of initial hemoglobin with birthweight (−23.6 g birthweight per 1 g/dl increase in hemoglobin concentration [$p<0.01$] and a 0.96 percent increase in the rate of birthweight under 2,500 g for each increase of 1 g/dl of initial hemoglobin [$p<0.05$]) (Rush et al., 1988). When these results were reexamined more closely for this report, there was no evidence of adverse relationship between a hemoglobin level under 10 g/dl or over 14 g/dl with adverse perinatal outcomes among whites. Among blacks, high hemoglobin (>14 g/dl) was associated with low birthweight in both first and second trimester participants, and low hemoglobin (<10 g/dl) was associated with low birthweight in first trimester participants, but numbers were small. For the much larger group of second trimester participants, there was no association of low hemoglobin with low birthweight (D. Rush, Tufts University, personal communication, June 1993).

The committee's opinion, based on the findings presented above and the information cited in the references to this report, is that the measures now in place are successfully addressing the problem of iron deficiency anemia among infants and young children. The preliminary finding that the prevalence of iron deficiency anemia is somewhat higher among children in one Hispanic subgroup, if confirmed, suggests a time lag in effectively reaching groups made up of recent immigrant populations. In the case of women, the prevalence of iron deficiency anemia persists at a level of 4 to 10 percent, and better information is needed to know why this is so. There is a need, in general, to have better data on specific population groups to define meaningful cutoff points for iron deficiency anemia in people of different racial and ethnic groups and to target interventions more effectively. These needs are further explained in the section on recommendations for research at the end of the committee's report.

Implications of Research on Excess Iron Intake

A recent article by Salonen and colleagues (1992) has renewed interest in the role of iron in chronic disease. In the study of Salonen and colleagues, the central question was relatively straightforward: Is excess body iron, as indicated by the plasma ferritin concentration, a significant positive risk factor for myocardial infarction? The committee determined that it would be necessary to review the role of iron in relation to chronic disease (cancer, atherosclerosis, and neurodegenerative disorders) postulated as resulting from excess iron through iron-catalyzed, biologically undesirable reactions. The information considered by the committee in pursuit of this question is contained in the paper by committee member John L. Beard, which appears in Appendix C to this report.

The committee determined that data are insufficient for a satisfactory test of the hypothesis of Salonen et al. (1992) in the U.S. population or to link excess iron intake to an increased risk of other chronic diseases. A follow-up analysis of NHANES I data (Sempos et al., under review) found no increased relative risk of myocardial infarction associated with excessive dietary iron intake or high levels of transferrin saturation, hemoglobin, or hematocrit (serum ferritin concentration were not measured) in people of all age, gender, and ethnic groups that were studied. Other analyses (Cooper et al., 1993; Daviglus et al., 1993; Dunn et al., 1993; Rimm et al., 1993; Stampfer et al., 1993) reached essentially the same negative conclusion.

In addition to the potential direct effects of high dietary iron intakes, large doses of supplemental iron may have an effect on the levels of other minerals (i.e., zinc, manganese, and copper) in plasma. Although there is a substantial research base on the interaction between iron and other minerals, it remains uncertain whether recommendations for the use of supplemental iron for the prevention of iron deficiency anemia may have a significant effect on other minerals consumed in the diet or taken in the form of supplements for other purposes (see Appendix B).

Developing Recommended Screening and Intervention Guidelines

The committee wishes to emphasize that the draft guidelines developed through its deliberations and contained in this report are based on current recommendations of expert groups for preventing and treating iron deficiency anemia among the populations under study (AAP, CON, 1993; IOM, 1990b, 1992b; LSRO, 1989), the collective expertise and experience of the committee's members, and its review of the scientific literature. The committee was not charged with nor had the resources to systematically evaluate the guidelines it produced for the screening, prevention, and treatment of iron deficiency anemia in this report as part of its program of work. Because the CDC plans to use the committee's draft recommendations to develop guidelines for public health clinics and clinicians in private practice nationwide, the committee recommends that the proposed procedure be evaluated, particularly with respect to costs and benefits, before implementation in the public and private sectors.

Such standards for basic requirements for screening have recently been outlined by Rush (1993) for a proposed nationwide screening program for the elderly.

1. Any screening procedure must have an acceptable level of sensitivity and specificity relative to some definite diagnostic procedure. Sensitivity (the ability to identify true cases) is important when an undetected case might have dire consequences, such as irreversible damage to the individual. Specificity (the ability of the screening procedure to classify correctly those without the condition) is important to avoid labeling someone with an incorrect presumptive diagnosis (false positive). Such false-positive diagnoses might both overburden the health care system and cause unnecessary anxiety, worry, expense, and bother for individuals who are not at risk.
2. The screening procedure for a *presymptomatic* diagnosis (as opposed to case finding for symptomatic disease) must give an adequate advantage in time (the lead time) over waiting for the individual to appear for care because of symptoms.
3. There must be a proven therapy for the disorder, and earlier treatment (the lead time) must confer benefits over treatment at the time symptoms might otherwise have led to presentation for care.
4. Finally, individual screening and therapy must offer benefits—both for the public health and the nation's economy—over other possible strategies such as universal or community prevention programs.

The committee believes that the research base for the hematologic tests suggested in its recommended guidelines for screening, prevention, and treatment of iron deficiency anemia meet the above criteria.

Additional standards for evaluating the committee's recommended guidelines are found in recent reports by the Institute of Medicine's Division of Health Care Services (IOM, 1990a, 1992a). The Committee on Clinical

Practice Guidelines has produced several reports on the development and evaluation of clinical practice guidelines. The committee recommends that the draft guidelines proposed in this report be further evaluated by the CDC against the eight attributes for clinical practice guidelines recommended by that Committee on Clinical Practice Guidelines (see Table 3-1 in that committee's full report [IOM, 1992a]).

Intervention Strategies: Efficacy and Safety

The methods for delivering iron to children and women can be categorized as either population based or as medicinal or therapeutic. The present population-based approach has two components—providing education to promote the consumption of iron-rich foods and increasing the iron content of the food supply. The therapeutic approach for delivering iron is through the voluntary or prescribed use of supplemental iron preparations.

Enrichment and Fortification

Enrichment of white bread and flour with iron (among other nutrients) is mandatory when the term *enrichment* is used in labeling and fortification of both standardized and nonstandardized foods has taken place. Fortification of ready-to-eat cereals gradually has increased, with many products now supplying 45 percent or more of the U.S. Recommended Daily Allowance for iron in a 1-ounce (28-g) serving, the amount required for a cereal to be eligible for purchase with food vouchers distributed in the U.S. Department of Agriculture's Special Supplemental Food Program for Women, Infants, and Children (WIC). The WIC program is targeted to low-income infants, children, and pregnant and lactating women, but it appears to have had the unintended effect of increasing the iron contents of products purchased by the broad array of consumers. The extent to which fortification of cereals with iron may have contributed to the increasing ferritin levels of men or the lower prevalence of anemia in the general population of young children is unknown.

Fortification with iron of foods consumed solely by infants—formula and infant cereals—allows for a clearly targeted intervention and is judged to have been effective. Appendix D outlines the trends in consumption of iron from the above sources, the current regulatory framework for enrichment and fortification, and the use and efficacy of iron-fortified infant cereals and meat in delivering iron to infants and children.

Education and Dietary Change

The most prevalent example of nutrition education for dietary change is embodied in the publication *Nutrition and Your Health: Dietary Guidelines for*

Americans (DHHS/USDA, 1991). Although there is no recommendation specific to iron, the first guideline, "Eat a Variety of Foods," specifically discusses ways to increase dietary consumption of iron through the consumption of iron-rich foods. The use of the dietary guidelines has become a universal component of all nutrition education programs. However, changes in diet brought about by educational efforts alone are very difficult to evaluate and quantify. Program evaluations generally neglect to include an examination of dietary change (Dwyer, 1982). Also, most evaluations are related to a combination of nutrition education and the delivery of food or supplemental iron—nutrition education and supplemental food (food stamps, WIC, or school lunch) or nutrition education and iron supplements (WIC, prenatal intervention studies [CDC-Ohio intervention in progress]).

A study of the dietary intake of preschool-age children showed that those who were provided supplemental food and nutrition education through the WIC program had significantly higher intakes of energy, ascorbic acid, and iron than nonparticipants (Brown and Tieman, 1986). Data from the 1985 National WIC Evaluation showed that program participants had significantly higher intakes of thiamin, niacin, vitamin B_6, ascorbic acid, and iron than nonparticipants (Rush et al., 1988). However, there was no residual long-term impact on dietary intake resulting from earlier enrollment in the program.

Supplementation for Infants and Children

It appears that the use of nonfood supplemental iron is generally unnecessary for most infants and children. However, supplemental iron as ferrous sulfate drops is recommended for preterm infants who are fed breast milk. Iron-fortified infant formula supplies adequate iron for formula-fed preterm infants. Iron-fortified infant formula, iron-fortified infant cereal, and meat are good dietary sources of iron for infants and children (See also Appendix D).

It appears that supplemental iron for infants is safe at prescribed doses. However, all supplemental iron preparations should be kept out of the reach of children to avoid poisoning. (See Appendix B for additional information.)

Supplementation for Women

Recommendations for the prescription of iron supplements have little prospect for success in preventing iron deficiency anemia unless they are accompanied by compliant behavior. Research shows that compliance is generally very inconsistent even for relatively simple drug regimens (Haynes et al., 1979). Although drug compliance is often poor even for individuals with life-threatening conditions such as diabetes, epilepsy, and organ transplantation, research shows that compliance is worse when the individual has no obvious illness, such as hypertension. The observed compliance with supplemental iron regimens is poor and is often worse among those who were initially anemic (Bonnar et al., 1969). Additionally, suspected poor compliance attributed to the side effects of supplemental iron has been disputed in studies in which only small differences in side effects were found among subjects taking therapeutic doses of iron (high doses of >180 mg of iron per day) and those taking placebos (Hallberg et al., 1967; Sölvell, 1970).

On the other hand, the proportion of the adult population that uses self-supplementation with over-the-counter mineral or vitamin-mineral products has increased from about 20 percent in the 1970s (Block et al., 1988) to about 40 percent of adults at present (Bender et al., 1992). In 1986, one in four women in the 18- to 44-year-old age group reported use of a supplement (most supplements taken were multivitamin-mineral supplements that contain iron), with a median dosage equal to 100 percent of the Recommended Dietary Allowance (RDA) (Stewart et al., 1985; Moss et al., 1989). Self-supplementation was higher among white women than among black and Hispanic women. It is not known whether users take the supplements regularly or intermittently.

Safety

Great caution should be exercised in storing iron-containing supplements. The composition of iron supplements intended for use by other household members (primarily women) is reported to be the most common cause of pediatric poisoning deaths in the United States. A toxic dose of elemental iron is 30 mg/kg of body weight for infants and children, and doses as low as 60 mg/kg have proved fatal (CDC, 1993).

RECOMMENDED GUIDELINES FOR PREVENTION, DETECTION, AND MANAGEMENT OF IRON DEFICIENCY ANEMIA

The committee's background papers and discussions provided the basis for developing its recommended guidelines for the prevention, detection, and management of iron deficiency anemia (previously published guidelines for the prevention, detection, and management of iron deficiency anemia are presented in Table 2; see also Appendixes B, C, and D). The sections below present the committee's guidelines for screening and treating iron deficiency anemia among infants, children, and nonpregnant and pregnant women of childbearing age. For all populations, the committee prefers and recommends dietary sources of iron over supplemental sources when possible, because food has physiological factors that improve iron absorption and other factors beneficial to overall health (NRC, 1989). In this report, dietary sources of iron include meat; iron-fortified infant formula; iron-fortified infant cereals; and iron-forti-

TABLE 2 Summary of Previously Published Guidelines to Prevent or Treat Iron Deficiency Anemia Among Infants, Children, and Nonpregnant and Pregnant Women of Childbearing Age

	Population				Women of Childbearing Age	
	Infants					
Source	Preterm	Term	Children	Adolescents	Nonpregnant	Pregnant
American Academy of Pediatrics[a]	2–3 mg/kg/day from ferrous sulfate drops (breastfed) Iron-fortified infant formula (nonbreastfed)	2–3 mg/kg/day from ferrous sulfate drops (breastfed; at age 4 to 6 mo.)[b] Iron-fortified infant formula (nonbreastfed)	Iron-fortified infant cereal (at age 4 to 6 mo.)	—	—	—
American College of Obstetricians and Gynecologists	—	—	—	—	—	Vitamin–mineral supplement (meeting RDA for pregnancy)
Canadian Paediatric Society	Supplemental iron for low-birth-weight infants (at age 8 wk–12 mo)	Iron-fortified infant formula (nonbreastfed) Iron-fortified infant cereal (breastfed)	—	—	—	—
Institute of Medicine	—	—	—	—	Well-balanced diet	30 mg/day for nonanemic 60–120 mg/day for anemic

Source						
Life Sciences Research Office	—	—	—	—	—	Routine iron supplementation for all pregnant women
Recommended Dietary Allowances, 10th ed.[d]	2 mg of supplemental iron per kg/day or iron-fortified infant formula	1 mg/kg/day (at age 0–3 mo) (nonbreastfed) 10 mg/day (at age 6 mo–3 yr)	10 mg/day (at age 3–10 yr)	12 mg/day, males; 15 mg/day, females	15 mg/day	30 mg/day from food sources and supplements
					60–180 mg of iron per day for mild anemia[c] 30 mg/day for continued follow-up treatment	
U.S. Preventive Services Task Force	Screen and, if necessary, treat No dosage recommended	—	—	—	Counsel on iron intake	Screen, and, if necessary, treat No dosage recommended[e]

[a] Recommended levels for all infants and children.
[b] Maintenance of breastfeeding beyond 6 months of age has been shown to protect against iron deficiency anemia in full-term infants.
[c] Nonanemic women do not require supplemental iron.
[d] Except for preterm infants and pregnant women, the source of iron is from the diet.
[e] A pending revision to the task force's statement on prevention of iron deficiency anemia during pregnancy recommends against routine iron supplementation during pregnancy (see Wolf and Washington, in press.).

SOURCES: AAP, CON (1969, 1976, 1985, 1989, 1992, 1993), ACOG (1989), Canadian Paediatric Society (1991), IOM (1990a,b, 1992b), LSRO (1991), NRC (1989), U.S. Preventive Services Task Force (1989).

fied, ready-to-eat cereals. However, for some specific populations, supplemental iron in addition to dietary sources is necessary.

Infants and Children

Although iron deficiency anemia appears to be continuing to decrease in prevalence among infants and children, there remain significant portions of the population at risk for developing iron deficiency anemia. For infants and children less than 6 years of age, anemia is defined as a hemoglobin concentration of less than 11.0 g/dl or a hematocrit level of less than 33 percent. Blacks may normally have lower hemoglobin levels; this justifies the use of cutoff values of less than 10.7 g/dl or less than 32 percent, respectively (Johnson-Spear and Yip, in press). Screening should be delayed if there is an indication of infection or if there has been an infection within the past 2 weeks.

For preterm infants who are no longer receiving hospital-based care, the committee recommends, after screening for anemia at no later than 3 months of age, the provision of supplemental iron (as ferrous sulfate drops) at 2 mg/kg/day or iron-fortified formula at no later than 1 month of age and continuing through 12 months of age to prevent further diminution of low fetal iron stores. Infants fed iron-fortified infant formula do not need an additional source of iron. Preterm infants should be screened for anemia by determining their hemoglobin or hematocrit level.

For most breastfed term infants, the committee recommends that they receive a source of iron (iron-fortified infant cereal, meat, or supplemental iron at 1 mg/kg/day) beginning at 4 months of age. After weaning from the breast, supplemental iron should stop being delivered and dietary sources of iron and iron-fortified formula should be used until the child is 12 months of age.

For formula-fed infants, the committee recommends the use of an iron-fortified infant formula until the infant consumes solid food or until age 12 months. When starting solid foods for all infants, iron-fortified infant cereal or meat should be used. Dietary counseling and nutrition education should include recommendations about the use of ascorbic acid-rich foods and meat to enhance iron absorption.

Term infants who are breastfed or non-breastfed infants who are not receiving iron-fortified infant formula should be screened for anemia at 9 months of age. For infants determined to be anemic, the infant should be placed on supplemental iron or iron-fortified formula. In the case of mild anemia in a formula-fed infant (hemoglobin level between 10 and 11 g/dl, or hematocrit level between 30 and 33 percent), an iron-fortified infant formula without supplemental iron drops may be adequate. All anemic infants should be reevaluated after 4 weeks of treatment. If there is a response of greater than or equal to 1 g/dl in the hemoglobin level or greater than or equal to a rise of 3 units in the hematocrit level or a value within the normal range, iron should be continued for 2 more months and then the source of supplemental iron should be discontinued. If there is no response or a response of less than 1 g/dl in the hemoglobin level or less than 3 units in the hematocrit level, the clinician should check for compliance with supplemental iron or determine the serum ferritin concentration. A serum ferritin concentration of greater than 15 µg/liter suggests that the anemia is not due to iron deficiency.

Infants with moderate or severe anemia (hemoglobin of <10.0 g/dl or hematocrit of <30 percent [<9.7 g/dl or <29 percent, respectively, for blacks]) should be evaluated by a physician.

For young children 2 years of age and older, no routine screening is needed if the child was not found to be anemic during earlier screenings. Children at mid-youth (6–12 years) with other risk factors (e.g., poverty, abuse, or poor household conditions) may need to be rescreened. As with the committee's earlier discussion of the consequences of excess iron and in the absence of research that indicates that iron deficiency anemia is a problem in adolescent boys, the committee cannot recommend a routine screening during childhood and adolescence. For adolescent girls, clinicians should follow the committee's recommendations for nonpregnant women of childbearing age.

Nonpregnant Women of Childbearing Age

The committee believes that some subpopulations of nonpregnant women of childbearing age (those in poverty, recent immigrants, etc.) are at special risk of developing iron deficiency anemia. The committee recommends that all nonpregnant women of childbearing age be screened for anemia at least once between 15 and 25 years of age. If other biologic risk factors for anemia are present (i.e., high menstrual blood loss, frequent blood donation, high parity) or there is a previous diagnosis of iron deficiency anemia, more frequent screening is warranted (i.e., every 2–3 years).

The anemia screening should be done with blood obtained by venipuncture. If anemia was suspected on the basis of a skin puncture sample, anemia should be confirmed with a repeat screen with blood obtained by venipuncture. For nonsmoking women, the committee recommends the following cutoff values: hemoglobin, <12.0 g/dl; hematocrit, <36 percent; or serum ferritin concentration, <12 µg/liter. A serum ferritin concentration determination is recommended to confirm iron deficiency anemia. Note that cutoff hemoglobin values for blacks should be set at 0.8 g/dl lower than the hemoglobin values given above. (See table of adjustments for smoking and altitude in the screening guidelines for nonpregnant women of childbearing age later in the report and in Appendix B.)

The recommended treatment approaches for iron deficiency anemia in nonpregnant women of childbearing age follow. If the concentration of hemoglobin is no more than 2 g/dl below the cutoff value for hemoglobin, the woman should be treated with a therapeutic dose of iron of about 60 mg twice a day (total daily dose of 120 mg of iron) and she should be provided with nutrition education (IOM, 1990b). The clinician should check for a response after 1 to 1.5 months. If there is no response (<1.0-g/dl increase in hemoglobin or <3-unit increase in hematocrit), despite what appears to be good compliance, the clinician should determine the serum ferritin concentration and consider other causes of anemia. A low hemoglobin or hematocrit level and a serum ferritin concentration of less than 20 µg/liter suggest iron deficiency anemia. In the presence of inflammation or infection, a low hemoglobin concentration or hematocrit level in conjunction with a serum ferritin concentration greater of than 15 µg/liter may also suggest iron deficiency anemia. If there has been a response resulting from supplemental iron, iron supplementation therapy should be continued until the hemoglobin concentration is 12.0 g/dl (see the table of adjustments for smoking and altitude in the screening guidelines for nonpregnant women of childbearing age later in the report), after which iron can be decreased to a maintenance level of about 30 mg of iron per day for 4 months and then discontinued.

Severe anemia is unusual in nonpregnant women of childbearing age and may not be due to iron deficiency. A complete medical history, including dietary history, a more thorough physical examination, and additional laboratory studies (i.e., complete blood count, reticulocyte count, and serum ferritin concentration), is indicated to determine the cause of anemia.

Alteration of diet may retard the development of iron deficiency anemia and avoid the need for supplemental iron in many nonpregnant women of childbearing age. Clinicians and other health care deliverers should emphasize dietary recommendations that encourage the consumption of ascorbic acid-rich foods or meats to enhance iron absorption from meals and discourage the consumption of tea or coffee with meals. In women at risk of multiple-nutrient deficiencies, clinicians may consider prescribing a multivitamin-mineral supplement of appropriate composition that contains approximately 30 mg of iron per tablet (see Appendix B, Table B-11, from IOM, 1992b).

Pregnant Women

The committee believes that pregnant women are the most at-risk population covered by this report. All pregnant women should be screened for iron deficiency anemia at the first prenatal visit and at least once during each subsequent trimester. Nutrition education about diet during pregnancy should be provided at every prenatal visit. This includes providing counseling on eating a diet rich in iron and foods that enhance iron absorption, avoiding foods that inhibit iron absorption (which should be consumed separately from iron-rich foods), and following guidelines in *Nutrition and Your Health Dietary Guidelines for Americans* (DHHS/USDA, 1991) and *Nutrition During Pregnancy and Lactation: An Implementation Guide* (IOM, 1992b).

The committee recommends that hemoglobin or hematocrit and, when feasible, serum ferritin concentration be determined early during the first trimester. Clinicians should refer the patient for further medical follow-up when the hemoglobin level is less than 9.0 g/dl or when the hemoglobin level is between 9.0 and 10.9 g/dl and the serum ferritin concentration is greater than 30 µg/liter. The committee does not recommend providing supplemental iron to pregnant women when the hemoglobin level is 11.0 g/dl or greater in the presence of a serum ferritin concentration greater than 20 µg/liter. When the hemoglobin level is between 9.0 and 10.9 g/dl and the serum ferritin concentration is between 12 and 20 µg/liter or the hemoglobin level is 11.0 g/dl or greater and the serum ferritin concentration is 20 µg/liter or less, 30 mg of supplemental iron should be provided on a daily basis.

The clinician should prescribe 60–120 mg of supplemental iron per day when the hemoglobin level is between 9.0 and 10.9 g/dl and the serum ferritin concentration is less than 12 µg/liter. Similar adjustments for hemoglobin and hematocrit levels in blacks should be made, as outlined above in the guidelines for nonpregnant women of childbearing age.

The hemoglobin level in anemic women should be evaluated at subsequent prenatal visits. If there has been no response to iron supplementation, the patient should be referred for additional follow-up. If the hemoglobin level is normal for that stage of pregnancy, the supplemental iron dose should be lowered to 30 mg/day.

If the first prenatal care visit does not occur until the second trimester, a blood specimen should be obtained by venipuncture and the hemoglobin level and serum ferritin concentration should be determined. Although the serum ferritin concentration declines during the second trimester of pregnancy, the measurement can be useful in assisting in the interpretation of the hemoglobin value. Clinicians should refer patients for further medical follow-up when the hemoglobin level is less than 9.0 g/dl. The clinician should prescribe 60–120 mg of supplemental iron per day when the hemoglobin level is between 9.0 and 10.4 g/dl and in the presence of a serum ferritin concentration of less than 12 µg/liter, and should prescribe 30 mg of supplemental iron per day when the hemoglobin level is 10.5 g/dl or greater in the presence of a serum ferritin concentration of 20 µg/liter or less. If the serum ferritin concentration is greater than 20 µg/liter, no intervention is recommended, regardless of the hemoglobin level.

At a visit during the third trimester, the clinician should obtain a blood specimen by venipuncture and determine the hemoglobin level. The patient should be referred for follow-up when the hemoglobin level is less than 9.0 g/dl. The clinician should prescribe 60–120 mg of supplemental iron per day when the hemoglobin level is between 9.0 and 10.9 g/dl and 30 mg of supplemental iron per day when the hemoglobin level is 11.0 g/dl or greater.

Supplemental iron can be stopped at the time of delivery unless anemia has continued throughout or after pregnancy or for those at high risk of iron deficiency anemia (i.e., excessive blood loss during pregnancy or multiple births). In that case, the clinician should continue supplementation until the 4- to 6-week postpartum visit. The committee's anemia criteria for nonpregnant women of childbearing age should be used for women at the 4- to 6-week postpartum visit.

Comments and Caution About Cutoff Values for Laboratory Tests

In this report, cutoffs for blood parameters are suggested in connection with recommended screening for iron deficiency. The committee emphasizes that it has selected cutoffs that should best be interpreted as follows: below this level, iron deficiency anemia may be present. For a significant proportion of people, the suggested cutoff levels do not mark any identified abnormality, and one should be careful to avoid generating unfounded concern in the patient or, in the case of infants, in the parents. Statistical evidence suggests that for a very substantial proportion of individuals selected for supplementation by the suggested cutoffs, a blood sample drawn a few days or weeks later (without any intervention) will show values in the normal range. However, for some individuals the values above the cutoffs will indicate a true anemia or iron deficiency. To protect those individuals, the committee made a conscious choice to set the cutoffs higher than might be used in clinical diagnostic practice, and certainly higher than the levels that are commonly recognized as driving clinical concern about detrimental consequences from iron deficiency anemia.

The recommendation to use lower cutoff values for hemoglobin in blacks in screening for iron deficiency anemia is consistent with the observation that hemoglobin values for this population are lower than those for other groups of comparable iron status (Johnson-Spear and Yip, in press; Perry et al., 1992). It is also consistent with the presently accepted definition of anemia as a hemoglobin concentration below the 95 percent confidence interval (i.e., below the 2.5th percentile) for a normal reference population. For all races, better information is urgently needed to provide functional, meaningful definitions of iron deficiency anemia and iron status.

Comments and Caution About Routine Use of Ferritin Values

Although the committee recommends the use of blood ferritin values as part of its screening protocol for the populations under study in this report, there are several explanatory comments and cautions about its use. It may be impractical or unfeasible to perform serum ferritin determinations in some settings. In settings where it is either impractical or too costly to obtain serum ferritin values, the committee continues to recommend the use of hemoglobin concentration or hematocrit value for the determination of iron deficiency anemia. When this is the case, clinicians and health care workers should be particularly aware that the anemia may not be the result of iron deficiency. However, the committee wishes to make it clear that it views serum ferritin values as being more precise in determining iron deficiency anemia. It also urges the development of more economical, uncomplicated serum ferritin concentration determination kits for use in many settings.

RECOMMENDED GUIDELINES FOR PREVENTING AND TREATING IRON DEFICIENCY ANEMIA IN INFANTS AND CHILDREN

A. Term, Breastfed Infants
1. Start a source of iron (supplemental iron at 1 mg/kg/day or iron-fortified infant cereal or meat) at age 4 months. If using supplemental iron, keep iron out of reach of infants and children.
2. After weaning from the breast, stop the iron supplement and use iron-fortified infant formula until age 12 months.
3. Avoid cow's milk until after age 12 months.

B. Term, Formula-Fed Infants
1. Use iron-fortified formula until age 12 months.
2. If feeding iron-fortified infant formula, iron-fortified cereal is not needed.
3. Avoid cow's milk until after age 12 months.

C. Preterm Infants (postdischarge from hospital care)
1. Start supplemental iron (2 mg/kg/day) or iron-fortified formula no later than age 1 month and continue to age 12 months.
2. Preterm infants (weight, >1,000 g) fed iron-fortified formula do not need additional iron.
3. For preterm breastfed infants, follow the recommended guidelines under A.2 through A.3 above.

D. Starting Solid Foods
1. After about age 4 months, use iron-fortified infant cereal and meat.
2. Use ascorbic acid-rich foods, meat, or both with meals to improve iron absorption.

E. Screen for Anemia by Determining Hemoglobin or Hematocrit
1. Screen term infants who are **not** receiving iron-fortified formula and breastfed infants (even those receiving an iron supplement, as a check on compliance) at age 9 months.
2. Screen preterm infants who are not receiving iron-fortified formula no later than age 3 months.
3. Delay screening if there is an infection or there has been an infection within the past 2 weeks.
4. Anemia (from ages 0.5 to 4.9 yr) is defined as hemoglobin of <11.0 g/dl or hematocrit of <33 percent. Blacks may normally have lower hemoglobin levels, justifying the use of cutoff values of <10.7 g/dl or <32 percent, respectively.

F. Treatment for Anemic Infants and Children

1. Infants with moderate or severe anemia, hemoglobin of <10.0 g/dl or hematocrit of <30 percent (<9.7 g/dl or <29 percent, respectively, for blacks), should be evaluated by a physician. For mild anemia, change to an iron-fortified formula or start iron drops at a dose of 3 mg of iron per kg/day. Keep iron supplements out of reach of children, because iron is a very common cause of poisoning in children.
2. After 4 weeks, check for a response consisting of a hemoglobin increase of 1 g/dl, a hematocrit increase of 3 percent, or a value within the normal range. If there is a response, continue iron drops (or iron-fortified formula) for 2 more months and then discontinue supplemental iron drops. Continue iron-fortified formula until age 12 months.
3. If there is no response, check compliance with supplemental iron regimen, determine serum ferritin concentration, or both. A serum ferritin concentration of >15 µg/liter suggests that the anemia is not due to iron deficiency.
4. Check hemoglobin or hematocrit again at age 15 or 18 months in infants who were found to be anemic at an earlier age. If there is a response, continue iron for 2 more months and then discontinue supplemental iron.

G. Children Over Age 24 Months

No routine screening is needed if the child was not anemic during prior screenings. However, children at mid-youth may need screening if other risk factors exist—poverty, abuse, poor household conditions, etc. In the absence of research findings that indicate that iron deficiency anemia is a problem in adolescent boys, the committee cannot recommend a routine screening for anemia during childhood and adolescence. See guidelines for preventing and treating iron deficiency anemia in nonpregnant women of childbearing age for information on screening adolescent girls.

RECOMMENDED GUIDELINES FOR PREVENTING AND TREATING IRON DEFICIENCY ANEMIA IN NONPREGNANT WOMEN OF CHILDBEARING AGE

A. General Screening of Women of Childbearing Age
1. All nonpregnant women should be screened for anemia between 15 and 25 years of age.
2. Consider screening once every 5 to 10 years if there are no risk factors for anemia. If medical or social risk factors for anemia are present (high parity, frequent blood donation, high menstrual blood loss, previous diagnosis of iron deficiency anemia, poverty, or recent immigration), more frequent screening is warranted.

B. Anemia Screening Procedure, if Necessary
1. Obtain blood by venipuncture. If anemia was suspected on the basis of a skin puncture sample, confirm analysis on venipuncture blood.
2. Use appropriate cutoff values for anemia as follows:

Parameter	Nonsmokers	10–20 cigs./day	21–40 cigs./day	Altitude >5,000 ft
Hemoglobin (g/dl)	12.0	12.3	12.5	12.5
Hematocrit (percent)	36.0	37.0	37.5	37.5

NOTE: Cutoff values for black women may normally be 0.8 g/dl lower than the hemoglobin values given above.

C. Counseling and Preventive Therapeutic Measures for Nonanemic Women
1. Most women do not require an iron supplement.
2. Women planning a pregnancy and at increased risk of iron deficiency anemia can take an iron-folate combination supplement containing folate at 0.4 mg/day and iron at about 30 mg/day.
3. In women with increased risk of nutrient deficiencies, consider a multivitamin-mineral supplement of appropriate composition that contains about 30 mg of iron.
4. Iron-containing supplements are best taken between meals or at bedtime with water or juice, not with tea, coffee, or milk. Keep out of reach of children, because iron is a very common cause of poisoning in children.

D. Treatment for Anemic Women
1. Mild anemia. If the concentration of hemoglobin is no more than 2 g/dl below the cutoff value (<10.0 g/dl), treat with a therapeutic dose of iron of about 60 mg twice a day (total daily dose, 120 mg). Provide dietary advice. Check for a response after 1 to 1.5 months. If there has been no response (an increase of at least 1.0 g/dl in hemoglobin or 3 percent in hematocrit), despite what appears to be good compliance, determine the serum ferritin con-

centration and consider other causes of anemia. Anemia and a serum ferritin concentration of <15 µg/liter suggest iron deficiency. If there has been a response, continue the therapeutic dose of iron for 2–4 months or until the hemoglobin concentration is 12.0 g/dl. After that time, the dosage of iron can be reduced to about 30 mg of iron per day for 6 months. A repeat serum ferritin concentration within normal limits is recommended prior to termination of iron therapy to determine repletion of iron stores.
2. Blacks may normally have slightly lower hemoglobin values than other races (0.8 g/dl less, on average). Anemia combined with a serum ferritin concentration of <15 µg/liter suggests iron deficiency. If the ferritin concentration is higher, the anemia is unlikely to be due to iron deficiency.
3. Severe anemia is unusual and may not be due to iron deficiency. Further history, including dietary history, a more thorough physical exam, and additional laboratory studies (i.e., complete blood count, reticulocyte count, and serum ferritin concentration) are indicated to determine the cause of anemia.

E. Advise on Diet
Eat a varied diet and enhance iron absorption by including meat, ascorbic acid-rich foods (fruit juice or fruit), or both in meals. Avoid tea or coffee with meals.

RECOMMENDED GUIDELINES FOR PREVENTING AND TREATING IRON DEFICIENCY ANEMIA IN PREGNANT WOMEN

A. Screen for Anemia at the First Prenatal Visit and Treat as Appropriate

1. If the first prenatal visit occurs in the first trimester, draw blood and determine hemoglobin and ferritin concentrations. Obtain medical evaluation when the hemoglobin concentration is <9.0 g/dl or the hemoglobin is between 9.0 and 10.9 g/dl and the serum ferritin concentration is >30 µg/liter.
2. Do not treat with iron when the hemoglobin concentration is ≥11.0 g/dl and the serum ferritin concentration is >20 µg/liter.
3. Give 30 mg of supplemental iron when the hemoglobin concentration is between 9.0 and 10.9 g/dl and the serum ferritin concentration is between 12 and 20 µg/liter, or the hemoglobin concentration is ≥11.0 g/dl and the ferritin concentration is ≤20 µg/liter.
4. Give 60–120 mg of supplemental iron when the hemoglobin concentration is between 9.0 and 10.9 g/dl and the ferritin concentration is <12 µg/liter.
5. At subsequent prenatal visits, evaluate the hemoglobin concentration. If there has been no response to iron supplementation, refer for additional medical evaluation. If the hemoglobin concentration is normal for that stage of pregnancy, lower the supplemental iron dose to 30 mg of iron per day.

NOTE: Blacks may normally have hemoglobin levels 0.8 mg less than those for other races. Adjustments should be made for higher hemoglobin levels observed in women accustomed to higher altitudes or those who smoke cigarettes.

B. Screen for Anemia at the Second-Trimester Visit and Treat as Appropriate

1. At a scheduled second-trimester visit, or if the first prenatal visit occurs in the second trimester, obtain a blood specimen and determine the hemoglobin and serum ferritin concentrations. Although the serum ferritin concentration declines during the second trimester of pregnancy, the measurement can be useful in assisting with the interpretation of the hemoglobin value. Refer for additional medical evaluation when the hemoglobin concentration is <9.0 g/dl.
2. Prescribe 60–120 mg of supplemental iron per day when the hemoglobin concentration is between 9.0 and 10.4 g/dl in the presence of a serum ferritin concentration of <12 µg/liter.
3. Prescribe 30 mg of supplemental iron per day when the hemoglobin concentration is ≥10.5 g/dl in the presence of a serum ferritin concentration of ≤20 µg/liter. If the serum ferritin concentration is >20 µg/liter, no treatment is needed.

4. Stop supplemental iron at delivery (at the 4- to 6-week postpartum visit if anemia continued through the third trimester).

C. Screen for Anemia at the Third-Trimester Visit and Treat as Appropriate

1. At a scheduled third-trimester visit, or if the first prenatal visit occurs in the third trimester, obtain a blood specimen and determine the hemoglobin concentration. Obtain medical evaluation when the hemoglobin concentration is <9.0 g/dl.
2. Prescribe 60–120 mg of supplemental iron per day when the hemoglobin concentration is between 9.0 and 10.9 g/dl.
3. Prescribe 30 mg of supplemental iron per day when the hemoglobin concentration is ≥ 11.0 g/dl.
4. Stop supplemental iron at delivery (at the 4- to 6-week postpartum visit if anemia continued through the third trimester).

D. Screen High-Risk Women for Anemia at the 4- to 6-Week Postpartum Visit

Screen women at high risk for iron deficiency anemia at the 4- to 6-week postpartum visit (risk factors include anemia continued through the third trimester, excessive blood loss during delivery, or multiple births). Obtain a blood specimen and determine the hemoglobin concentration. Interpret the results with the same criteria as for nonpregnant women.

E. Advise on Diet at Each Prenatal Visit

1. Eat a varied diet of iron-rich foods and foods that enhance iron absorption (meats and ascorbic acid-rich fruits). Items that inhibit absorption of iron (tea, coffee, whole-grain cereals [particularly bran], unleavened whole-grain breads, and dried beans) should be consumed separately from iron-rich foods.
2. Follow the guidelines of *Nutrition and Your Health: Dietary Guidelines for Americans* (DHHS/USDA, 1991) and *Nutrition During Pregnancy and Lactation: An Implementation Guide* (IOM, 1992b).

NOTE: If 120 mg of supplemental iron per day is prescribed, recommend delivery of one 60-mg tablet twice a day.

RECOMMENDATIONS FOR RESEARCH

In conducting its critical review of the available information related to public health approaches to the prevention, detection, and management of iron deficiency anemia, the committee identified two major gaps in the research base. The first consists of information on the efficacy of routine iron supplementation during pregnancy and the second consists of several gaps in the research base for public policy decisionmaking.

Efficacy of Routine Iron Supplementation During Pregnancy

The evidence on which to base a coherent policy of whether to routinely provide iron supplements for iron deficiency to pregnant women who are not overtly anemic—and if so, at what stage of pregnancy supplementation should begin and at what dosage—is unclear. Almost all observational studies that have related hemoglobin or hematocrit to birth weight or duration of gestation have shown a consistent U-shaped relationship with adverse outcome at very low (<8 or 9 g/dl) or high (>13 g/dl) hemoglobin levels. These relationships are true for hemoglobin measured at any time during pregnancy, but are weakest for the relationship between a low hemoglobin concentration in the third trimester and an adverse outcome (i.e., premature birth, low birthweight).

The meaning of these observations is further obscured because, taken in toto, there has been no observed effect of iron supplementation on the duration of gestation or birth weight in rigorous controlled trials (Hemminki and Starfield, 1978).

Thus, it is unclear whether an adverse perinatal outcome associated with the level of hemoglobin, low or high, can be reversed by iron supplementation or some other intervention.

High levels of hemoglobin have consistently been observed in association with a severely adverse perinatal outcome. Those who advocate universal supplementation posit that high levels of hemoglobin have little or nothing to do with iron status but rather to a unphysiologically low level of expansion of plasma volume during pregnancy. However, this has not been studied directly. Taylor and Lind (1979) demonstrated that iron supplementation has no effect on plasma volume. They found that although the red blood cell mass increased by 180 ml among controls, it increased by 349 ml among those treated with 65 mg of elemental iron daily. Thus, the hemoglobin concentration was increased, and therefore, it is unclear whether hemoglobin levels could also be raised among women with inadequate plasma volume expansion and whether it would possibly cause problems associated with a high hemoglobin concentration. Also, among women who received supplemental iron in controlled trials of iron supplementation during pregnancy, the weighted value of the mean plus two standard deviations for the hemoglobin concentration closest to term (between 36 and 40 weeks) was 14.6 g/dl (Table 3). This concentration is well above that

TABLE 3 Mean Reported Hemoglobin Level Closest to Term Among Iron-Supplemented Women

Hemoglobin Concentration (g/dl) (mean ± SD)	Mean ± 2 SD	No. of Subjects	Week of Gestation	Reference
12.4 ± 0.94[a]	14.3	49	37	Chanarin and Rothman, 1971
12.4 ± 0.86[a]	14.1	24	36	Svanberg et al., 1976
13.2 ± 1.2	15.6	16	40	Puolakka et al., 1980
12.7 ± 0.8	14.3	21	36	Taylor et al., 1982
12.6 ± 0.8	14.3	22	37–40	Romslo et al., 1983
12.8 ± 1.2	15.2	21	40	Wallenburg and van Eijk, 1984
12.4 ± 1.35[a]	15.1	16	38	Dawson and McGanity, 1987
Weighted[b] mean	14.63			

NOTE: See Table B-2 in Appendix B. SD is standard deviation.

[a] Calculated from authors' data.
[b] Weighted by number of subjects.

associated with an adverse perinatal outcome and suggests the possibility that routine supplementation may possibly induce dangerous hemoglobin concentrations. It has been assumed that supplementation only affects those with low hemoglobin values and that there will not be an increase in hemoglobin concentration in those with high or fairly high hemoglobin concentrations (i.e., that there is a truncated distribution with supplementation: low values would increase, but higher values would not). On the other hand, all of the studies presented change in terms of mean and standard deviation (or standard error) and did not present any distributional data to test the assumption that there is little or no increase in high values.

Thus, a nested set of assumptions underlies a policy of routine supplementation, and all of these assumptions need to be tested by objective and careful research. The first assumption is that the adverse outcomes associated with high hemoglobin concentrations have little or nothing to do with red blood cell mass but, rather, are a function of contracted or inadequately expanded plasma volume. This assumption needs testing in an observational study that asks the following: Are high hemoglobin concentrations with adequately expanded plasma volume associated with an adverse outcome, or are only high hemoglobin concentrations associated with inadequately expanded plasma volume?

The second assumption that needs explicit study is whether routine supplementation with iron produces a change only among those with lower hemoglobin levels or affects the entire range of the distribution. If the latter is true, does it affect women with inadequately contracted plasma volume in ways that may result in hemoglobin concentrations that could be dangerous?

Finally, these preliminary studies need to be the basis for a large, well-designed, randomly controlled trial of routine iron supplementation in women who do not have frank iron deficiency anemia in early pregnancy. Without such a study, it cannot be concluded from data currently published in observational or experimental studies that iron supplementation is beneficial to the progress of pregnancy and that it presents no dangers to the pregnancy or in the perinatal period. So far there is little or no evidence that routine iron supplementation is of benefit to fetal growth, to the duration of pregnancy, or to indices other than the replenishment of the iron stores of the mother (not the infant). Moreover, by 6 weeks postpartum, hemoglobin levels in women who do not receive iron supplements are, on average, at their prepregnancy levels.

The need for caution is reflected by a new expert committee's report that concludes that iron supplementation for women who do not have iron deficiency anemia is unnecessary (Woolf and Washington, in press). This is, however, the conclusion of a minority of clinicians in the United States, where iron supplementation of pregnant women has been routine for years.

Without benefit of further research, the committee believes that the current routine iron supplementation practice should not be changed. **The committee believes that the standard practice of routine iron supplementation during pregnancy should not be altered without evidence as firm as that required** to initiate some new medical intervention or practice. The fact that iron supplementation during pregnancy has been routine in the United States for decades does not provide a body of evidence that it is, overall, advantageous; the support for the practice is based on an extrapolation from an incomplete database.

Research Base for Public Policy

Improved Data on Iron in the Food Supply

To more accurately determine the impact of iron fortification on dietary intake, **the committee recommends improvement in the database on the types of iron used to fortify foods, the quantity of iron added to those foods, and the iron usage patterns by population subgroups (race, gender, and income and in relation to patterns of serum ferritin concentrations).** Once the database is improved, researchers will be better equipped to estimate the iron intakes of various population subgroups. Such estimates, perhaps with the addition of projections based on recent trends, can form the basis for future recommendations for iron fortification of foods. Such data will be particularly useful for predicting which populations of consumers, if any, are at risk of excessive iron intake. Similar data also should be collected on over-the-counter supplement preparations and their use.

Expand the Sample of Infants and Minorities in National Nutrition Surveys

In preparing its screening guidelines for infants, the committee relied on NHANES data for children 2 through 5 years of age. Estimates and extrapolations for infants based on data on preschool-age children are probably not appropriate for the screening recommended at 9 months of age. In the future, **nutrition surveys should include a sufficient number of infants in the survey sample size to permit estimates of iron deficiency anemia for groups of infants at 3-month age intervals from birth through 2 years of age.** These data are needed to determine the appropriate cutoff values for infants with different ethnic and racial backgrounds.

Because of the differences in iron nutrition status among racial and ethnic subgroups, **nutrition surveys should include larger numbers of individuals from ethnic subgroups in survey samples.** For example, the sample used in NHANES III for the "Hispanic" population covers only Mexican Americans. Larger samples of Hispanic and other ethnic groups could be added to future survey samples (e.g., Cubans, Puerto Ricans, and those from the Caribbean). By expanding the representation of ethnic subgroups in national nutrition surveys, more data would be available to correlate dietary beliefs and practices with health status measurements.

More Information on the Prevalence of Iron Deficiency Anemia Among Adolescents

Another group for which prevalence data on iron deficiency anemia were lacking is adolescents. **The committee recommends that more information be collected about the prevalence of iron deficiency anemia in adolescent males and females and about the critical determinants of iron nutrition during adolescence.** Intervention programs that are designed to work for older women or poor and underprivileged mothers stand a good chance of not working for teens because of social issues pertinent only to adolescence. For adolescent males, more information on the effect of iron intake and athletic performance and endurance is needed.

New Determinants of Iron Deficiency Anemia in the First Trimester of Pregnancy

A key issue confronting the committee was the ability of clinicians and public health practitioners to identify early in pregnancy women who are at risk for developing iron deficiency anemia in the first trimester of pregnancy. Data from Scholl and colleagues (1992) indicate that the first trimester is a time of great risk for the developing fetus, with the potential for iron deficiency anemia to have a negative impact on fetal growth. **The committee therefore recommends that studies be done to identify new determinants of iron deficiency anemia in pregnant women during the first trimester of pregnancy.**

Conduct Cost-Benefit Studies on the Use of Serum Ferritin Concentration Determinations

Costs vary widely for the laboratory test to determine serum ferritin concentration. This is primarily based on the fact that different settings apply different overhead costs to the charge associated with this test. Administration of the basic test generally costs less than $1. The committee has recommended that laboratory determination of serum ferritin concentration be conducted to confirm the presence of iron deficiency anemia. This laboratory test is currently used in many settings as part of the prenatal laboratory profile conducted throughout the course of pregnancy. Although there is substantial agreement on the value of the use of the serum ferritin concentration determination to confirm iron deficiency anemia, at present there are few cost-benefit data to support the widespread use of the test. Additionally, the number of individuals who would benefit from this additional screening tool is not entirely clear. Therefore, **the committee recommends that cost-benefit studies be conducted to determine the value of the widespread use of serum ferritin concentration tests as part of the screening protocol for evaluating iron deficiency anemia.**

Sensitivities and Specificities of New Tests to Measure Iron Status

Although the state of the science for determining iron status has improved markedly, **the committee recommends that more information be collected on the sensitivities and specificities of new tests for iron status, particularly in relation to different prevalences of iron deficiency anemia among at-risk population groups.** For example, little information is available on the distribution of ferritin and transferrin receptors among different ethnic and racial groups. There is a need for expanded information on the predictive value of iron tests for specific at-risk groups (i.e., ferritin receptor).

Alternative Approaches to the Prevention and Detection of Iron Deficiency Anemia

Lastly, the committee found little information about the cost-benefit attributes of alternative public health approaches for preventing and detecting iron deficiency anemia. **Therefore, the committee recommends that more information be collected about the costs and benefits of alternative approaches for preventing and detecting iron deficiency anemia.** There is little information in the literature about the efficacy or effectiveness of alternative intervention strategies, and the committee therefore did not find it surprising that little information is available on the cost-benefit attributes of alternative public health approaches. Some straightforward studies on the cost implications of policy changes in the types of laboratory tests used to evaluate iron nutrition and the presence of iron deficiency anemia should be undertaken. Similarly, analyses of the cost implications of policy changes related to changes in cutoff values should also be conducted. The cost and effectiveness of ready-to-eat cereal fortification versus other methods of increasing iron should be of interest to WIC officials in particular. Trends in consumption patterns for major food classes should be monitored. Changes in food selection in response to dietary guidelines to reduce fat and increase nutritional quality—that is, to increase consumption of whole-grain cereals, vegetables, and beans and to decrease intake of red meat—may affect an individual's overall intake of iron, heme iron, and bioavailability (owing to the intake of phytate and other factors). Analysis of data from the 1987–1988 Nationwide Food Consumption Survey showed a weak but statistically significant negative correlation between diet quality variables defined as percentage of energy from fat and intakes of 15 nutrients below two-thirds of the Recommended Dietary Allowance. This led the authors to conclude that the adults surveyed seldom choose diets that are both high in nutrients and low in fat (Murphy et al., 1992).

REFERENCES

AAP, CON (American Academy of Pediatrics, Committee on Nutrition). 1969. Iron balance and requirements in infancy. Pediatrics 43:134–142.
AAP, CON (American Academy of Pediatrics, Committee on Nutrition). 1976. Iron supplementation for infants. Pediatrics 58:765–768.
AAP, CON (American Academy of Pediatrics, Committee on Nutrition). 1985. Nutritional needs of low-birth-weight infants. Pediatrics 75:976–986.
AAP, CON (American Academy of Pediatrics, Committee on Nutrition). 1989. Iron-fortified infant formulas. Pediatrics 84:1114–1115.
AAP, CON (American Academy of Pediatrics, Committee on Nutrition). 1992. The use of whole cow's milk in infancy. Pediatrics 89:1105–1109.
AAP, CON (American Academy of Pediatrics, Committee on Nutrition). 1993. Pediatric Nutrition Handbook. Elk Grove, Ill.: American Academy of Pediatrics.
ACOG (American College of Obstetricians and Gynecologists). 1989. Committee on Professional Standards. Standards for Obstetric-Gynecological Services, 7th ed. Washington, D.C.: ACOG.
Bender, M.M., A.S. Levy, R.E. Schucker, and E.A. Yetley. 1992. Trends in prevalence and magnitude of vitamin and mineral supplement usage and correlation with health status. J. Am. Diet. Assoc. 92:1096–1101.
Block, G., C. Cox, J. Madans, G.B. Schreiber, L. Licitra, and N. Melia. 1988. Vitamin supplement use by demographic characteristics. Am. J. Epidemiol. 127:297–309.
Bonnar, J., A. Goldberg, and J.A. Smith. 1969. Do pregnant women take their iron? Lancet 1:457–458.
Brown, J.E., and P. Tieman. 1986. Effect of income and WIC on the dietary intake of preschoolers: Results of a preliminary study. J. Am. Diet. Assoc. 86:1189–1191.
Canadian Paediatric Society, Nutrition Committee. 1991. Meeting the iron needs of infants and young children: An update. Can. Med. Assoc. J. 144:1451–1453.
CDC (Centers for Disease Control). 1989. CDC criteria for anemia in children and childbearing-aged women. Morbid. Mortal. Weekly Rep. 38:400–404.
CDC (Centers for Disease Control and Prevention). 1993. Toddler deaths resulting from ingestion of iron supplements—Los Angeles. Morbid. Mortal. Weekly Rep. 42(6):111–113.
Chanarin, I., and D. Rothman. 1971. Further observations on the relation between iron and folate status in pregnancy. Br. Med. J. 2:81–84.
Cook, J.D., B.S. Skikme, and R.D. Baynes. 1993. Serum transferrin receptor. Annu. Rev. Med. 44:63–74.
Cooper, R.S., and Y. Liao. 1993. Iron stores and coronary heart disease: Negative findings in the NHANES I Epidemiologic Follow-up Study. Circulation 87:686 abstract 33.

Daviglus, M.L., A.R. Dyer, K. Liu, R.B. Shekelle, and J. Stamler. 1993. Is hemoglobin a risk factor for CHD? Circulation 87: abstract.

Dawson, E.B., and W.J. McGanity. 1987. Protection of maternal iron stores in pregnancy. J. Reprod. Med. 32:478–487.

DHHS/USDA (U.S. Department of Health and Human Services and U.S. Department of Agriculture). 1991. Nutrition and Your Health: Dietary Guidelines for Americans, 3rd ed. Washington, D.C.: U.S. Government Printing Office.

Dunn, J.E., K. Liu, A. Dyer, and J. Serwitz. 1993. Physical activity and occupation in young employed black and white men and women: The CARDIA study. Circulation 87: abstract.

Dwyer, J.T. 1982. Food for thought on food stamps. Am. J. Public Health 72:786.

Ferguson, B.J., B.S. Skigne, K.M. Simpson, R.D. Baynes, and J.D. Cook. 1992. Serum transferrin receptor distinguishes the anemia of chronic from iron deficiency anemia. J. Lab. Clin. Med. 119:385–390.

Hallberg, L., L. Ryttinger, and L. Sölvell. 1967. Side effects of oral iron therapy: A double-blind study of different iron compounds in tablet form. Acta Med. Scand. Suppl. 459:3–10.

Haynes, R.B., D.W. Taylor, and D.L. Sackett, eds. 1979. Compliance in Health Care. Baltimore: Johns Hopkins University Press.

Hemminki, E., and B. Starfield. 1978. Routine administration of rion and vitamins during pregnancy: Review of controlled clinical trials. Br. J. Obstet. Gynaecol. 85:404–410.

IOM (Institute of Medicine). 1990a. Clinical Practice Guidelines: Directions for a New Program. Report of the Committee to Advise the Public Health Service on Clinical Practice Guidelines, Division of Health Care Services. Washington, D.C.: National Academy Press.

IOM (Institute of Medicine). 1990b. Nutrition During Pregnancy. Report of the Committee on Nutrition During Pregnancy and Lactation, Food and Nutrition Board. Washington, D.C.: National Academy Press.

IOM (Institute of Medicine). 1992a. Guidelines for Clinical Practice: From Development to Use. Report of the Committee on Clinical Practice Guidelines, Division of Health Care Services. Washington, D.C.: National Academy Press.

IOM (Institute of Medicine). 1992b. Nutrition During Pregnancy and Lactation: An Implementation Guide. Report of the Subcommittee for a Clinical Applications Guide, Committee on Nutrition During Pregnancy and Lactation, Food and Nutrition Board. Washington, D.C.: National Academy Press.

Johnson-Spear, M.A., and R. Yip. In press. Hemogobin difference between black and white women with comparable iron status: Justification for race-specific criteria? Am. J. Clin. Nutr.

Kim, I., D.W. Hungerford, R. Yip, S.A. Kuester, C. Zyrkowski, and F.L. Trowbridge. 1992. Pregnancy Nutrition Surveillance System—United States, 1979–1990. CDC Surveillance Summaries. Morbid. Mortal. Weekly Rep. 41(No. SS-7):26–42.

LSRO (Life Sciences Research Office). 1984. Assessment of the Iron Nutritional Status of the U.S. Population Based on Data Collected in the Second National Health and Nutrition Examination Survey, 1976–1980. Bethesda, Md.: Federation of American Societies for Experimental Biology.

LSRO (Life Sciences Research Office). 1989. Nutrition Monitoring in the United States—An Update Report on Nutrition Monitoring. DHHS Publication No. (PHS) 89-1255. Public Health Service. Washington, D.C.: U.S. Government Printing Office.

LSRO (Life Sciences Research Office). 1991. Guidelines for the Assessment and Management of Iron Deficiency in Women of Childbearing Age. Bethesda, Md.: Federation of American Societies for Experimental Biology.

Moss, A.J., A.S. Levy, I. Kim, and Y.K. Park. 1989. Use of vitamin and mineral supplements in the United States: current users, types of products, and nutrients. Advance Data from Vital and Health Statistics. volume:174.

Murphy, S.P., D. Rose, M. Hudes, and F.E. Viteri. 1992. Demographic and economic factors associated with dietary quality for adults in the 1987–1988 Nationwide Food Consumption Survey. J. Am. Diet. Assoc. 92:1352–1357.

NRC (National Research Council). 1989. Recommended Dietary Allowances, 10th ed. Report of the Subcommittee on the Tenth Edition of the Recommended Dietary Allowances, Food and Nutrition Board, Commission on Life Sciences. Washington, D.C.: National Academy Press.

Perry, G.S., T. Byers, R. Yip, and S. Margen. 1992. Iron nutrition does not account for hemoglobin differences between blacks and whites. J. Nutr. 122:1417–1424.

Puolakka, J., O. Jänne, A. Pakarinen, and R. Vihko. 1980. Serum ferritin as a measure of stores during and after normal pregnancy with and without iron supplements. Acta Obstet. Gynecol. Scand. Suppl. 95:43–51.

Rimm, E., A. Ascherio, M.J. Stampfer, G.A. Colditz, E. Giovannucci, and W.C. Willett. 1993. Dietary iron intake and risk of coronary disease among men. Circulation 87:692 (abstract P22).

Romslo, I., K. Haram, N. Sagen, and K. Augensen. 1983. Iron requirements in normal pregnancy as assessed by serum ferritin, serum transferrin saturation, and erythrocyte protoporphyrin determinations. Br. J. Obstet. Gynaecol. 90:101–107.

Rush, D. 1993. Evaluating the Nutrition Screening Initiative. Am. J. Public Health 83:944–945.

Rush, D., J. Leighton, N.L. Sloan, J.M. Alvir, D.G. Horvitz, W.B. Seaver, G.C. Garbowski, S.S. Johnson, R.A. Kulka, J.W. Devore, M. Holt, J.T. Lynch, T.G. Virag, M.B. Woodside, and D.S. Shanklin. 1988. The National WIC Evaluation: Evaluation of the Special Supplemental Food Program for Women, Infants, and Children. VI. Study of infants and children. Am. J. Clin. Nutr. 48(Suppl.):484–511.

Salonen, J.T., K. Nyyssönen, H. Korpela, J. Tuomilehto, R. Seppänen, and R. Salonen. 1992. High stored iron levels are associated with excess risk of myocardial infarction in eastern Finnish men. Circulation 86:803–811.

Scholl, T.O., M.L. Hediger, R.L. Fischer, and J.W. Shearer. 1992. Anemia vs. iron deficiency: Increased risk of preterm delivery in a prospective study. Am. J. Clin. Nutr. 55:985–988.

Sempos, C.T., A.C. Looker, R.F. Gillum, and D.M. Maycuk. Under review. Body iron stores and coronary heart disease incidence and mortality from selected causes. N. Engl. J. Med.

Sölvell, L. 1970. Oral iron therapy-side effects. Pp. 573–583 in L. Hallberg, H.G. Harwerth, and A. Vannotti, eds. Iron Deficiency: Pathogenesis, Clinical Aspects, Therapy. London: Academic Press.

Stampfer, M.J., F. Grodstein, I. Rosenberg, W. Willett, and C. Hennekens. 1993. A prospective study of plasma ferritin and risk of myocardial infarction in U.S. physicians. Circulation 87:688 abstract P7.

Stewart, M.L., J.T. McDonald, A.S. Levy, R.E. Schucker, and D.P. Henderson. 1985. Vitamin and mineral supplement use: A telephone survey of adults in the United States. J. Am. Diet. Assoc. 85:1585–1590.

Svanberg, B., B. Arvidsson, A. Norrby, G. Rybo, and L. Sölvell. 1976. Absorption of supplemental iron during pregnancy—A longitudinal study with repeated bone-marrow studies and absorption measurements. Acta Obstet. Gynecol. Scand. Suppl. 48:87–108.

Taylor, D.J., and T. Lind. 1979. Red cell mass during and after normal pregnancy. Br. J. Obstet. Gynaecol. 86:364–370.

Taylor, D.J., C. Mallen, N. McDougall, and T. Lind. 1982. Effect of iron supplementation on serum ferritin levels during and after pregnancy. Br. J. Obstet. Gynecol. 89:1011–1017.

Wallenburg, H.C.S., and H.G. van Eijk. 1984. Effect of oral iron supplementation during pregnancy on maternal and fetal iron status. J. Perinat. Med. 12:7–11.

Woolf, S.H., and A.E. Washington. In press. Routine supplementation of iron during pregnancy: Summary of the evidence. Review by the U.S. Preventive Services Task Force. J. Am. Med. Assoc.

Yip, R., N.J. Binkin, L. Fleshood, and F.L. Trowbridge. 1987a. Declining prevalence of anemia among low-income children in the United States. J. Am. Med. Assoc. 258:1619–1623.

Yip, R., K.M. Walsh, M.G. Goldfarb, and N.J. Binkin. 1987b. Declining prevalence of anemia in childhood in a middle-class setting: A pediatric success story? Pediatrics 80:330–334.

Appendixes

A
Acknowledgments

Molly Anthony, Bureau of Maternal and Child Health, Health Resources and Services Administration, Public Health Service, U.S. Department of Health and Human Services

Sandra J. Bartholmey, Nutrition Services, Gerber Products Company, Fremont, Michigan

Fergus Clydesdale, Department of Food Science, University of Massachusetts at Amherst

James R. Connor, Department of Neurosciences, Hershey Medical Center, Hershey, Pennsylvania

Alta Engstrom, Nutrition Services, General Mills, Inc., Minneapolis, Minnesota

Sara B. Fein, Consumer Studies Branch, Division of Market Studies, Office of Scientific Analysis and Support, Food and Drug Administration, Public Health Service, U.S. Departement of Health and Human Services

Suzanne Harris, Nutrition Foundation, International Life Sciences Institute, Washington, D.C.

Alan Heaton, Consumer Studies Branch, Division of Market Studies, Office of Scientific Analysis and Support, Food and Drug Administration, Public Health Service, U.S. Departement of Health and Human Services

Jan Lilja, Food and Nutrition Service, U.S. Department of Agriculture, Alexandria, Virginia

Anne C. Looker, National Center for Health Statistics, Centers for Disease Control and Prevention, Public Health Service, U.S. Department of Health and Human Services, Washington, D.C.

Abe Parvanta, Maternal and Child Health Branch, Division of Nutrition, National Center for Chronic Disease Prevention and Health Promotion, Centers for Disease Control and Prevention, Public Health Service, U.S. Department of Health and Human Services, Atlanta, Georgia.

Howard Riddick, Human Nuitrition Information Service, U.S. Department of Agriculture, Hyattsville, Maryland

Darryl Schaller, Science and Technology, Kellogg's, Inc., Battle Creek, Michigan

Richard Seifman, Office of Nutrition, U.S. Agency for International Development, Washington, D.C.

Elizabeth Yetley, Office of Special Nutritionals, Center for Food Safety and Applied Nutrition, Food and Drug Administration, Public Health Service, U.S. Department of Health and Human Services, Washington, D.C.

Ray Yip, Maternal and Child Health Branch, Division of Nutrition, National Center for Chronic Disease Prevention and Health Promotion, Centers for Disease Control and Prevention, Public Health Service, U.S. Department of Health and Human Services, Atlanta, Georgia.

B

Iron Deficiency Anemia: A Synthesis of Current Scientific Knowledge and U.S. Recommendations for Prevention and Treatment

Peter R. Dallman

Iron deficiency anemia is a relatively common nutritional problem in the United States, particularly among infants, adolescents, and women of childbearing age. Its prevention deserves a high priority because iron deficiency anemia has serious consequences, yet its prevalence can be substantially reduced at modest cost. There has been great progress in preventing iron deficiency anemia among infants and children, but the prevalence among pregnant women of childbearing age remains high. The purpose of this appendix is to provide a brief review of the characteristics of iron deficiency anemia and to review recent guidelines for its prevention in primary health care settings.

This appendix provided background information for the Committee on the Prevention, Detection, and Management of Iron Deficiency Anemia Among U.S. Children and Women of Childbearing Age of the Food and Nutrition Board, Institute of Medicine. It also incorporated revisions and additions suggested after review of the paper by the committee, but does not indicate universal concurrence with its content. The committee then developed summary guidelines for children, nonpregnant women of childbearing age, and pregnant women that are contained in the main report.

REVIEW OF KNOWLEDGE

Metabolism and Physiology

Iron in the Body

The total amount of iron in the body of an adult woman averages 2.3 g (Bothwell et al., 1979), about the weight of a dime. Figure B-1 shows the distribution of this iron, which is similar in women of reproductive age and in children. An average of about 85 percent of total body iron can be classified as essential because it serves well-defined physiologic functions. Essential iron

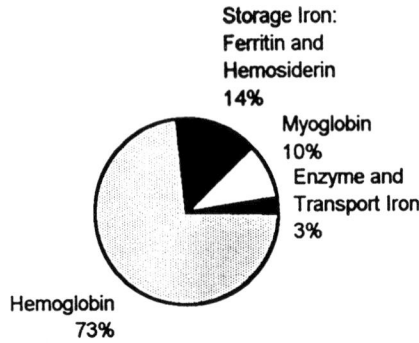

FIGURE B-1 Distribution of iron in women of childbearing potential (total body iron, 2.3 g—the weight of a dime). SOURCE: Values are from Table 1, p. 2, in Bothwell and Charlton (1981).

compounds include hemoglobin, which accounts for about three-quarters of total body iron and functions in the transport of oxygen from the lungs to tissues. Because hemoglobin circulates in the blood and accounts for a large proportion of essential body iron, its concentration often best reflects iron status. Other essential iron compounds include myoglobin, the red iron protein of muscle, and the mitochondrial iron proteins, which are essential for the oxidative production of cellular energy in the form of adenosine triphosphate. Iron deficiency is not associated with physiologic impairment until the production of essential iron compounds is diminished (Dallman, 1986).

A second category of iron compounds is referred to as storage iron. Storage iron compounds include ferritin and hemosiderin, which are present primarily in the liver, spleen, and bone marrow. They serve as a reserve that ensures an adequate supply of iron for the production of essential iron compounds, and they maintain body iron homeostasis by regulating the amount of iron absorbed from the diet. Storage iron is less abundant in women and children than in men: about 14 percent of total body iron, on average (Figure B-1), and about 25 percent, respectively. The serum ferritin concentration provides an estimate of storage iron reserves.

Iron Homeostasis

Body Iron Regulation Body iron is regulated primarily by modifying the percentage of food iron that is absorbed. Among healthy, nonpregnant women, body iron remains relatively stable, because the amount of iron absorbed each

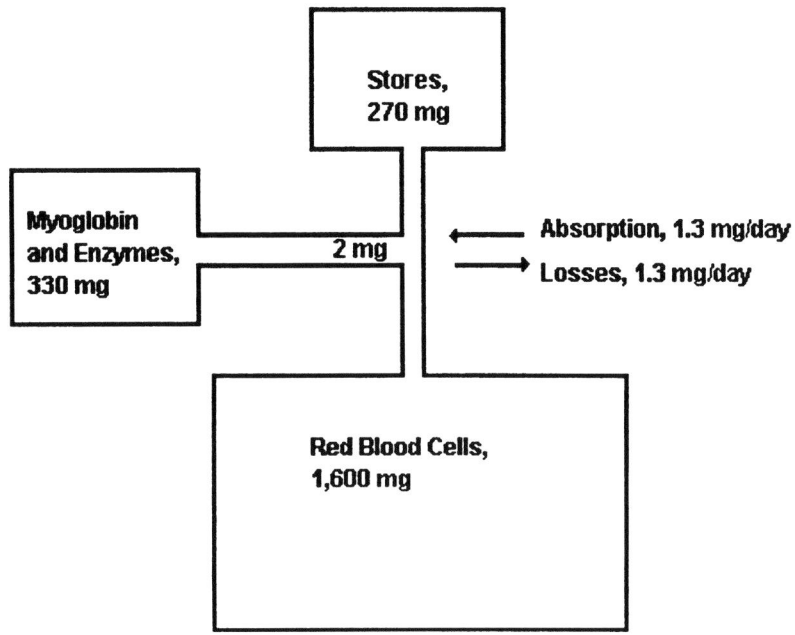

FIGURE B-2 Iron balance in women of childbearing potential. SOURCE: Based on Bothwell et al. (1979).

day is roughly equivalent to the amount of iron lost (Figure B-2) and is less than 0.05 percent of total body iron (Bothwell et al., 1979). Iron homeostasis is normally maintained because iron absorption is inversely proportional to the amount of storage iron. When storage iron decreases, as it does during pregnancy or rapid growth, iron absorption increases (Figure B-3). This homeostatic adaptation is greatest with diets containing high levels of available iron (Cook, 1990). Low iron stores per se indicate that an individual is vulnerable to developing iron deficiency anemia, but as long as the production of essential iron remains intact, there are no known physiologic handicaps from having low iron reserves (Dallman, 1986).

Iron Loss and Absorption Differences Between Women and Men Women have greater iron losses and absorb a greater percentage of iron from food than do men. During their childbearing years, women typically have less storage iron than men primarily because of menstrual blood loss (Bothwell et al., 1979). They compensate by absorbing, on average, about twice as much iron from the diet as men, 12 versus 6 percent (Table B-1).

Average menstrual blood loss is about 30 ml/month (Hallberg et al., 1966), but 10 percent of women regularly lose more than 80 ml/month (Figure B-4) and are likely to become anemic because their iron loss is usually greater than that which can be compensated for by increased absorption of iron from the

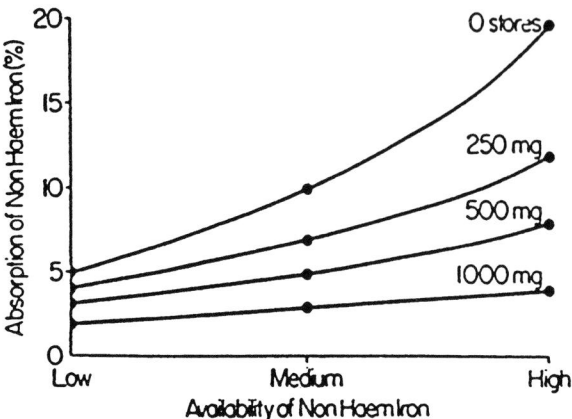

FIGURE B-3 Non-heme iron absorption from three different types of diets as the percent absorption of non-heme iron by individuals with no body iron stores and with 250-, 500-, and 1,000-mg iron stores. As iron stores decrease, the percentage of iron absorbed increases, helping to maintain homeostasis. This compensatory mechanism is less effective with diets of low iron bioavailability (common in developing countries) than with diets with medium and high levels of iron bioavailability, which are more typical in the United States. A daily diet of low iron bioavailability is one containing fewer than 30 g of meat, poultry, or fish (lean, raw weight) or less than 25 mg of ascorbic acid. The comparable figures for a diet of medium iron bioavailability are 30 to 90 g of meat, poultry, or fish or 25 to 75 mg of ascorbic acid, whereas a diet of high iron bioavailability is one containing more than 90 g of meat, poultry, or fish or more than 75 mg of ascorbic acid. Alternatively, it is one containing 30 to 90 g of meat, poultry, or fish plus 25 to 75 mg of ascorbic acid. SOURCE: Data from Monsen and coworkers (1978), in Bothwell et al. (1979).

diet. Unfortunately, such women are typically unaware of their high levels of blood loss. Consequently, the most practical way to identify them is by screening for anemia as part of a periodic health maintenance checkup (LSRO, 1991).

Menstrual blood loss varies with some methods of contraception (Figure B-5), roughly decreasing to half with oral contraceptives (the pill) and doubling with intrauterine devices (IUDs) (Bothwell and Charlton, 1981), Thus, inquiring about the method of contraception helps to predict the risk of iron deficiency; the risk is greatest in women who use an IUD.

Iron Needs During Pregnancy Pregnancy imposes increased iron needs for the growth of the fetus and for expansion of maternal blood volume (Hallberg, 1988; IOM, 1990a) (Figure B-6). Even women who are not iron deficient at the beginning of pregnancy (on the basis of the hemoglobin concentration) are at risk of developing an iron-responsive depression in hemoglobin concentration in the third trimester unless they receive supplemental iron (Table B-2). Among women who are already iron deficient when they become pregnant, the severity of the deficiency will usually increase as pregnancy progresses unless they take an iron supplement.

TABLE B-1 Iron Balance in Women Compared with That in Men

Iron Parameter	Women	Men
Total body iron, g	2.3	3.5
Storage iron, g	0.3	1.0
Food iron, mg/day	11	15
Iron absorption, percent	12	6
Iron absorption, mg/day	1.3	0.9
Iron loss, mg/day	1.3	0.9

SOURCE: Based primarily on data in Bothwell et al. (1979).

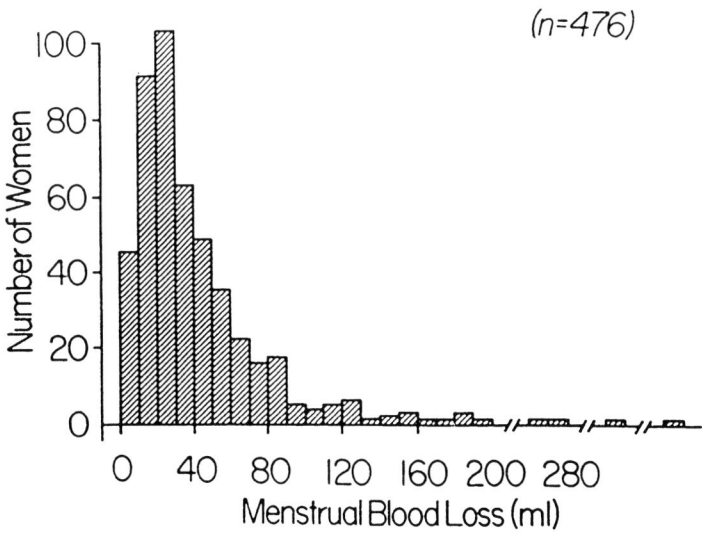

FIGURE B-4 Frequency distribution of menstrual blood loss. Although the mean menstrual blood loss is about 30 ml/month, about 10 percent of women lose more than 80 ml/month. SOURCE: Data from Hallberg et al. (1966), adapted from Bothwell et al. (1979).

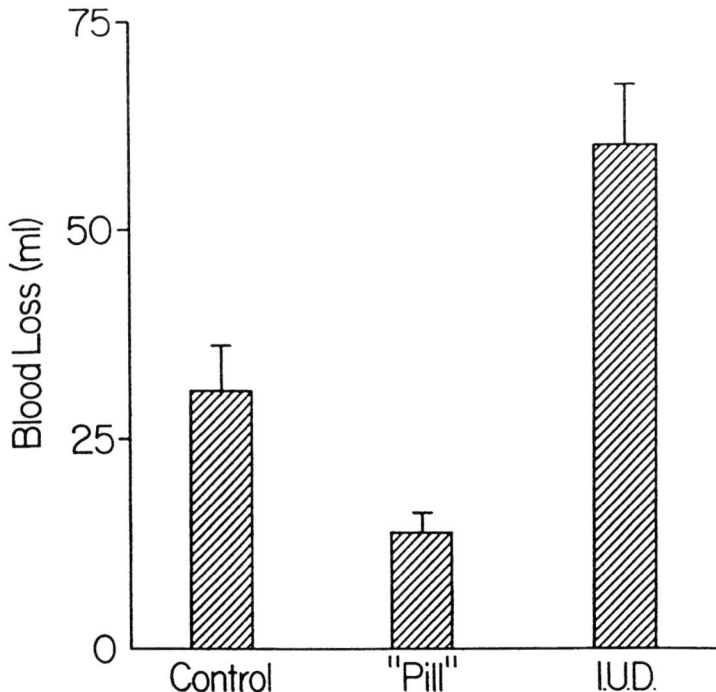

FIGURE B-5 Menstrual blood loss by method of contraception as mean ± standard deviation menstrual blood loss in three groups of women. The control group comprised normal women, the pill group comprised normal women taking the combination variety of oral contraceptives, and the IUD group comprised women using intrauterine devices (IUDs). SOURCE: Figure from Bothwell and Charlton (1981).

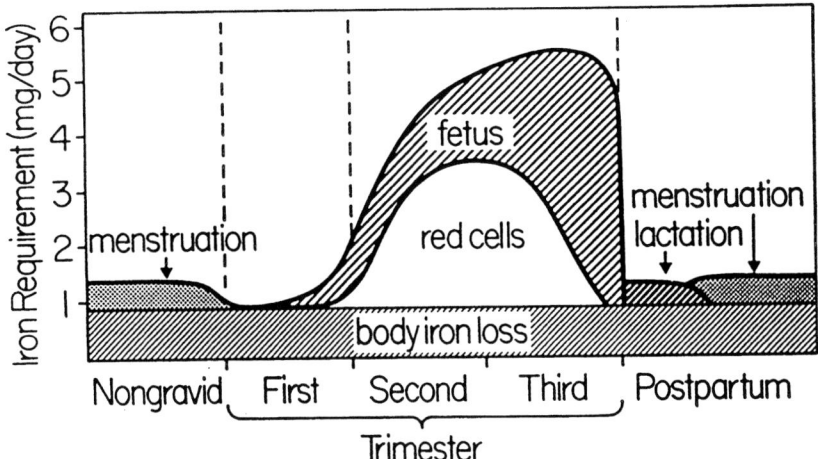

FIGURE B-6 Schematic representation of the need for absorbed iron during pregnancy. Iron requirements increase markedly during the second and third trimesters. SOURCE: From Bothwell et al. (1979).

TABLE B-2 Effects of Iron Supplementation on Mean Hemoglobin Concentration in Late Pregnancy

Dose of Elemental Iron[a]	Number of Subjects		Hemoglobin, g/dl, at 35–36 weeks of Gestation[b]			Reference
	Supplemented	Controls	Supplemented	Controls	Difference[b]	
30 mg/day as ferrous fumarate[c]	49	46	12.4	11.4	1.0	Chanarin and Rothman, 1971
100 mg, twice daily, with meals, sustained release	24	26	12.4	11.4	1.0	Svanberg et al., 1976
100 mg, twice daily, sustained release	16	16	12.7	11.0	1.7	Puolakka et al., 1980
65 mg (+ 350 μg of folate)	21	24	12.7	11.0	1.6	Taylor et al., 1982
200 mg/day	22	23	12.6	11.3	1.3	Romslo et al., 1983
105 mg, sustained release, at breakfast	21	23	12.6	12.2	0.4	Wallenburg and van Eijk, 1984
65 mg as part of multivitamin-mineral supplement after meals	16	13	12.4	11.4	1.0	Dawson and McGanity, 1987

[a] Ferrous sulfate, unless otherwise stated.
[b] All differences were statistically significant except for Wallenburg and van Eijk (1984).
[c] Doses of 60 and 120 mg did not result in higher hemoglobin values.

SOURCE: From IOM (1990b).

Iron Needs of Infants Among infants, iron needs are primarily for growth. A high hemoglobin concentration at birth and abundant neonatal iron stores protect most term infants against iron deficiency until 4 months of age (Dallman, 1988). Indeed, total body iron scarcely changes during this period because of the physiologic decline in hemoglobin concentration; iron stores also diminish by 4 months of age (Figure B-7). Term infants are at the greatest risk of developing iron deficiency between 4 and 12 months of age and subsequently, when the iron needs for rapid growth must be supplied by the diet. At 1 year of age, for example, iron absorption is about four times greater than excretion, the difference being used for growth (Figure B-8). The risk of developing iron deficiency anemia during this period depends largely on the diet (Penrod et al., 1990; Pizarro et al., 1991; Tunnessen and Oski, 1987). Although iron deficiency anemia is rare in infants receiving iron-fortified formula, it is common in those fed unfortified formula or cow's milk (Figure B-9). Cow's milk not only has an extremely low concentration of iron but it also results in increased fecal blood loss (Ziegler et al., 1990) (Figure B-10). Furthermore, the higher calcium content of cow's milk compared with that of breast milk contributes to poor iron absorption (Hallberg et al., 1992). Exclusively breastfed infants may also develop iron deficiency, but only after about 6 months of age (Calvo et al., 1992; Duncan et al., 1985; Pizarro et al., 1991; Siimes et al., 1984), if they are not given an iron supplement (Figure B-9).

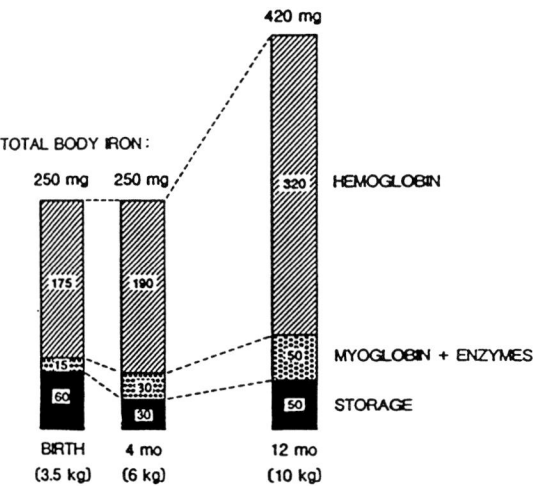

FIGURE B-7 Changes in body iron during infancy. There is little change in total body iron between birth and 4 months of age. In contrast, total body iron increases markedly during later infancy. The high iron needs from 4 to 12 months of age help to explain why the risk of iron deficiency is greatest during this period. SOURCE: Dallman (1988).

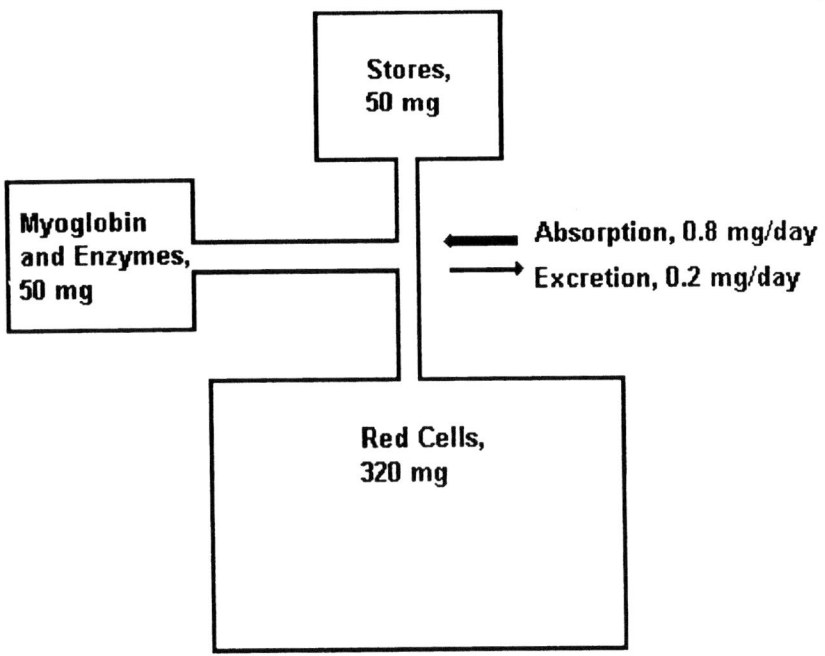

FIGURE B-8 Iron metabolism in the 1-year-old infant. Iron absorption must exceed iron loss to allow growth; however, daily iron absorption and loss, even in infancy, are normally a minute percentage of total body iron. MB + ENZ = myoglobin and enzyme iron. SOURCE: Reproduced with minor modifications from Dallman (1988), with permission from Hanley & Belfus.

In the United States, there has recently been a marked decline in the prevalence of iron deficiency anemia among infants and young children (Yip et al., 1987a,b). This improvement is attributable to concurrent changes in infant feeding practices that would be expected to improve iron nutrition, including less use of cow's milk in the first year of life, more use of iron-fortified formulas, and less use of low-iron formulas (Fomon, 1987). Iron absorption studies suggest (Fomon et al., 1989) and clinical trials indicate (Walter et al., 1993) that iron-fortified infant cereals also play a significant role in preventing iron deficiency anemia.

Low-birth-weight infants may become iron deficient after 2 months of age and possibly earlier unless they are given an iron supplement (Lundström et al., 1977; Siimes et al., 1984) (Figure B-11). Their iron needs are greater because of their lower neonatal stores, a more rapid relative growth rate, and often, blood loss resulting from the increased number of laboratory studies that their early care may require. For low-birth-weight infants fed human milk, supplemental iron is recommended to start at about 2 weeks of age at a dose of 2 to 3 mg of elemental iron per kg/day (AAP, CON, 1985). Infants fed iron-fortified formula usually obtain sufficient amounts of iron to make an additional supplement unnecessary.

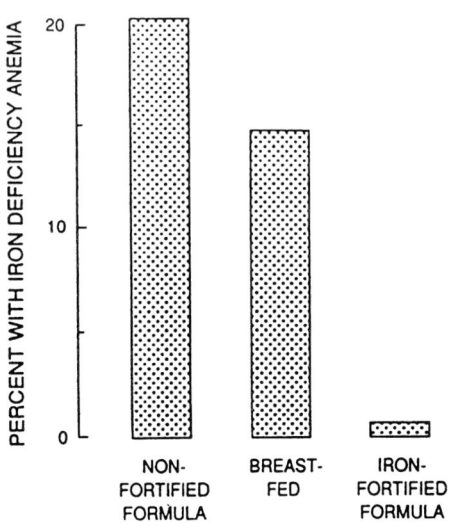

FIGURE B-9 Iron deficiency anemia among 9-month-old children who have been fed different diets. SOURCE: From Pizzaro et al. (1991).

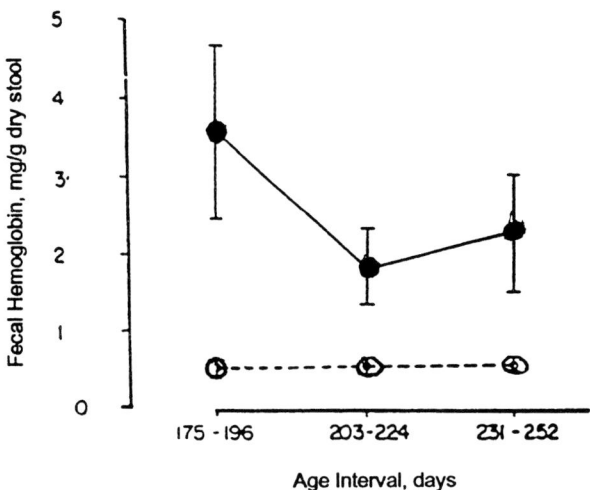

FIGURE B-10 The fecal hemoglobin concentrations of infants fed formula (•) and infants fed cow's milk (o) after 168 days of age. Early feeding of cow's milk to infants results in increased fecal blood loss. Bars indicate standard errors. SOURCE: Adapted from Ziegler et al. (1990).

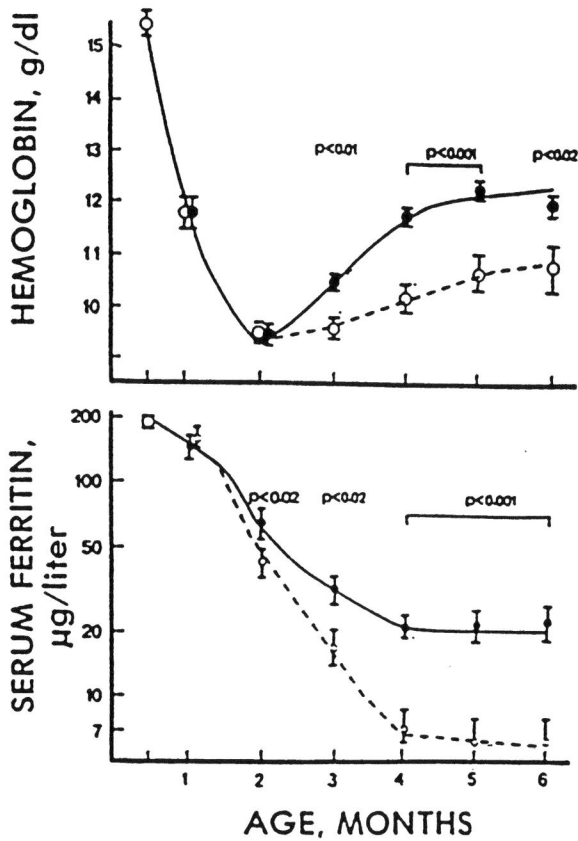

FIGURE B-11 Iron deficiency anemia among low-birth-weight infants. Low-birth-weight infants weighing 1,000 to 2,000 g are likely to develop iron deficiency anemia after 2 months of age if not given iron supplements (o). The supplemented infants (•) received a total of 2 mg of iron/kg/day as ferrous sulfate starting at 2 weeks of age. SOURCE: From Lundström et al. (1977).

Childhood and Adolescence After infancy, iron deficiency becomes less common (Yip et al., 1987a,b) as the rate of growth decreases and the diet becomes more diversified. During adolescence, however, the prevalence of iron deficiency rises again (LSRO, 1984) because iron needs increase with the adolescent growth spurt (Dallman, 1992) (Figure B-12). Presumably, iron deficiency is even more common among pregnant adolescents, in whom the iron needs for pregnancy follow closely after the increased needs for growth. However, no iron deficiency prevalence data for pregnant adolescents in the general population are available.

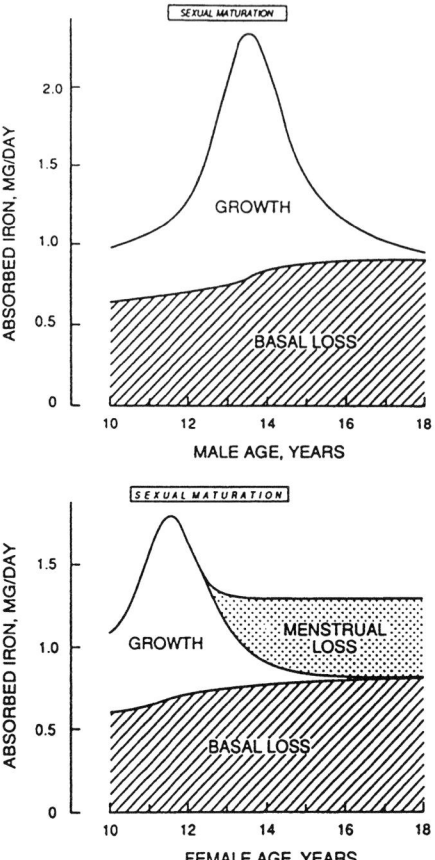

FIGURE B-12 Iron needs of male and female adolescents. There is an increase in the need for absorbed iron with the adolescent growth spurt, helping to account for an increased prevalence of iron deficiency at this age. The top of the figure is based on a representative male whose peak adolescent growth is at 13.5 years, near the average in the United States. Iron needs peak sharply during the growth spurt but decline rapidly thereafter. Sexual maturation (progression from Tanner stages 2 to 5) begins about 2 years before peak growth; this signals the period of greatest iron needs. The bottom of the figure is based on a representative female whose peak growth is at 11.5 years, near the average in the United States. Although iron needs rise to a maximum during peak growth, they remain high subsequently in females, since the iron needs to replace menstrual iron loss begin about 1 year after peak growth. SOURCE: Dallman (1992).

Absorption of Iron from Food The form of iron in the diet is even more important than the amount (Bothwell et al., 1989; Charlton and Bothwell, 1983; Cook et al., 1991; Hallberg, 1982; Hallberg and Rossander, 1982). Heme iron is better absorbed than non-heme iron, but non-heme iron makes up about 90 percent of the iron in the diet, and its absorption is strongly influenced by enhancers and inhibitors of iron absorption consumed in the same meal. These influences are greatest among individuals whose storage iron is depleted

(Figure B-13) (Cook, 1990). The diets of most people in the United States are relatively rich in the two most important enhancers, meat and ascorbic acid, and are therefore quite good sources of absorbable or bioavailable iron (LSRO, 1989) (Figure B-14). Phytates and polyphenols are important inhibitors. Protein, per se, has a highly variable influence on iron absorption, ranging from the facilitating effect of animal tissue protein (meat) to the strong inhibitory properties of isolated soy protein.

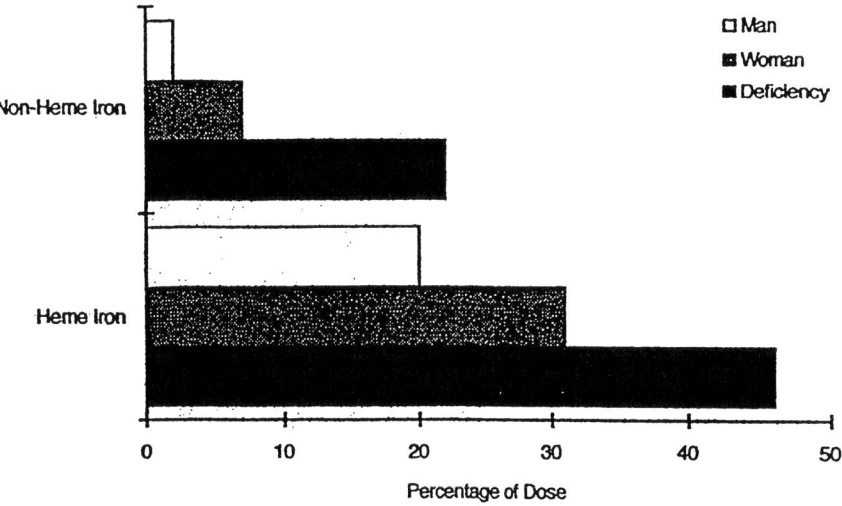

FIGURE B-13 Variation in absorption of heme and non-heme iron from a hamburger meal at different levels of iron status. Percent absorption from each form of iron is shown for an iron-replete man, a premenopausal woman, and a person with iron deficiency, individuals with assumed serum ferritin concentrations of 100, 30, and 10 µg/liter, respectively. SOURCE: From Cook (1990).

The beverage consumed with a continental breakfast has a major impact on the amount of iron absorbed from the entire meal (Figure B-15). Tea and coffee inhibit iron absorption when consumed with a meal, whereas orange juice and other sources of vitamin C (ascorbic acid) are major enhancers. There is less influence on iron absorption when these beverages are consumed between meals. Meals that contain inhibitors of iron absorption, such as polyphenols (tannins in tea and certain vegetables) or phytate (in whole-grain cereals), can nevertheless become good sources of absorbable iron if they also include ascorbic acid as an enhancer (Siegenberg et al., 1991). Along similar lines, Galan et al. (1991) found that, contrary to expectations, good calcium sources such as low-fat milk or yogurt did not significantly depress iron absorption when consumed with a meat-containing meal. Thus, nutritionally valuable foods that happen to inhibit iron absorption need not be avoided if the diet contains adequate enhancers of iron absorption.

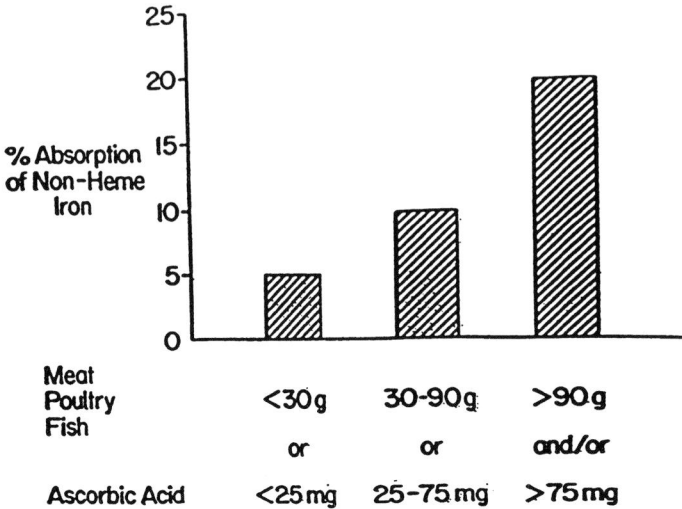

FIGURE B-14 Iron absorption as the percentage of iron absorbed from a diet varies according to the amount of the important enhancers of iron in the diet. The following estimates are based on the percent absorption of non-heme iron by individuals with no body iron stores from three different types of diets. A daily diet with *low iron bioavailability* is one containing less than 30 g of meat, poultry, or fish (lean, raw weight) or less than 25 mg of ascorbic acid. The comparable figures for a diet with *medium iron bioavailability* are 30 to 90 g of meat, poultry, or fish or 25 to 75 mg of ascorbic acid. A diet with *high iron bioavailability* is one containing more than 90 g of meat, poultry, or fish or more than 75 mg of ascorbic acid. Alternatively, it is one containing 30 to 90 g of meat, poultry, or fish plus 25 to 75 mg of ascorbic acid. Most diets in the United States are of medium to high iron bioavailability. SOURCE: Data from Monsen and coworkers (1978), in Bothwell and Charlton (1981).

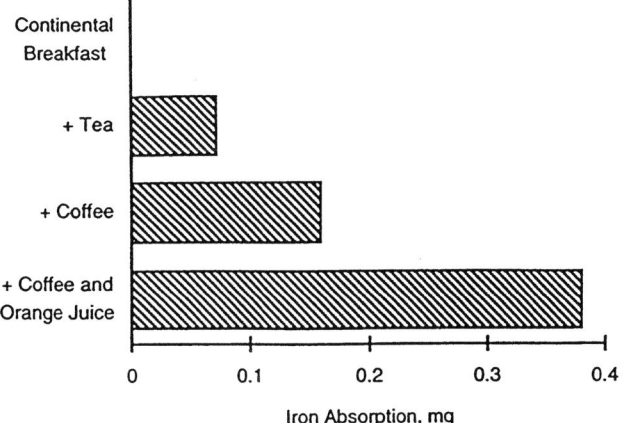

FIGURE B-15 Effect of beverage type on iron absorption. The beverage consumed with a meal (a continental breakfast, for example) has a large effect on the amount of iron absorbed from the entire meal. SOURCE: Data from Rossander et al. (1979), in Bothwell and Charlton (1981).

Cook and colleagues (1991) recently obtained results indicating that the magnitude of differences in non-heme iron bioavailability might be less than absorption studies of single meals would suggest, particularly among those who are not iron deficient. When non-heme iron absorption was measured from the whole diet over a 2-week period, the difference between an iron absorption-enhancing and an iron absorption-inhibitory diet was 2.5-fold. In contrast, data based on a single meal showed a much larger difference (5.9-fold). Similar questions were raised by an earlier study of long-term administration of ascorbic acid, which might have been expected to increase iron stores, but it appeared to have little or no effect on serum ferritin levels (Cook et al., 1984). It was concluded that in the context of the U.S. diet, the role of enhancers was less important than the role of inhibitors of non-heme iron absorption (Cook et al., 1991). This topic deserves further investigation, since it is highly relevant to providing advice on how to improve iron nutrition. More information is needed regarding the effectiveness of dietary intervention (decreasing the consumption of inhibitors and increasing that of enhancers of iron absorption in the diet in the treatment or prevention of iron deficiency anemia).

For adults and children 2 years of age and older, the guidelines in *Nutrition and Your Health: Dietary Guidelines for Americans* (DHHS/USDA, 1991) at present provide a basis for good general nutrition and iron nutrition. In addition, for enhancement of iron absorption from an entire meal in individuals at risk of iron deficiency, it is advisable to include a good source of ascorbic acid or meat, fish, or poultry as part of the meal. Beverages, like tea and coffee, that inhibit iron absorption are best consumed between meals.

Absorption of Iron from Iron-Fortified Foods Absorption of iron from iron-fortified foods has been a major factor in the declining prevalence of iron deficiency anemia among infants and children (Bothwell and MacPhail, 1992; Cook and Bothwell, 1984; Hurrell, 1992). Even the use of fortified cereal products, however, cannot be expected to prevent iron deficiency anemia among women of childbearing age who have unusually high menstrual blood losses (Swiss and Beaton, 1974). The impact of the iron fortification of cereal products on the iron nutrition of other women is unknown, but it may help to account for the relatively low prevalence of iron deficiency anemia, about 3 percent among nonpregnant white women, in the United States (LSRO, 1984).

Ferrous sulfate is commonly used to fortify infant formula and other products sold in cans and other airtight containers. Ferrous sulfate is also used to fortify bread and other bakery products that have a short shelf life. Since ferrous sulfate is highly soluble, it is as well absorbed as the intrinsic iron in these foods. However, compounds such as ferrous sulfate are not suitable for fortifying many foods that are marketed and stored for long periods in air-permeable packages, because most highly soluble forms of iron promote fat oxidation and rancidity. For this reason, elemental iron powders are commonly used to fortify such foods. The elemental iron powder used to fortify infant cereal contributes significantly to the prevention of iron deficiency anemia (Walter et al., 1993).

In Europe, the relatively nonreactive and insoluble ferric orthophosphate and ferric pyrophosphate are also widely used. There is less quantitative information about the effectiveness of these less well absorbed forms of iron used to fortify foods.

Absorption of Iron from Iron-Containing Supplements Absorption of iron from iron-containing supplements is influenced by the dose, the iron stores of the recipient, whether iron is taken with or between meals, and whether it is taken alone or as part of a vitamin-mineral supplement (IOM, 1990a). The percentage of iron absorbed is high at the lowest doses and decreases substantially as the dose is increased. This is an important factor for clinicians to bear in mind, particularly in the treatment of iron deficiency anemia, because compliance is likely to be impaired by the substantial prevalence of gastrointestinal side effects when doses are increased to greater than 120 mg/day. In general, iron absorption from supplements is greatest in iron-deficient individuals, because as mentioned above in respect to food iron, absorption is inversely proportional to iron stores.

Iron supplements are absorbed about twice as well when given between meals rather than with meals. It is also better to give an iron supplement with water or juice than with a beverage that is known to inhibit iron absorption, such as tea, coffee, or milk.

Slow-release iron supplements of various kinds have been developed to decrease the prevalence of side effects when large doses are used. These preparations are typically more expensive than commonly used, rapidly soluble forms of iron, such as ferrous sulfate, ferrous gluconate, and ferrous fumarate (Kastrup, 1992). When given with a meal, slow-release preparations may be better absorbed than ferrous sulfate, but they are less well absorbed under fasting conditions (Ekenved et al., 1976).

Women in their childbearing years commonly take iron as part of a vitamin-mineral tablet. Calcium and magnesium are the constituents of such tablets that are most likely to inhibit iron absorption (Babior et al., 1985; Seligman et al., 1983).

Definitions of Anemia, Iron Deficiency Anemia, and Iron Deficiency

Anemia

Anemia is defined as a hemoglobin concentration (or hematocrit) that is below the 95 percent range for healthy, well-nourished individuals of the same age, sex, and stage of pregnancy. Hemoglobin values are normally lower in children than in nonpregnant adults (Table B-3). During puberty, hemoglobin concentrations in males rise above those in females. During pregnancy, hemoglobin values gradually fall to a low point in the second trimester (Table B-4,

TABLE B-3 Hemoglobin and Hematocrit Cutoffs for Children, Nonpregnant Women, and Men[a]

Sex and Age (yr)	Hemoglobin, g/dl	Hematocrit, %
Both sexes		
0.5–4.9	11.0	33
5.0–11.9	11.5	35
Female		
≥12	12.0	36
Male		
12.0–14.9	12.5	37
15.0–19.9	13.0	38
≥ 20	13.5	41

[a] Hemoglobin values are rounded off to the nearest 0.5 g/dl, and hematocrit is rounded off to the nearest percent.

SOURCE: Data are based on fifth percentile values from the second National Health and Nutrition Examination Survey (NHANES II) after exclusion of individuals with a likelihood of being iron deficient (CDC, 1989) and the *Pediatric Nutrition Handbook* (AAP, CON, 1993).

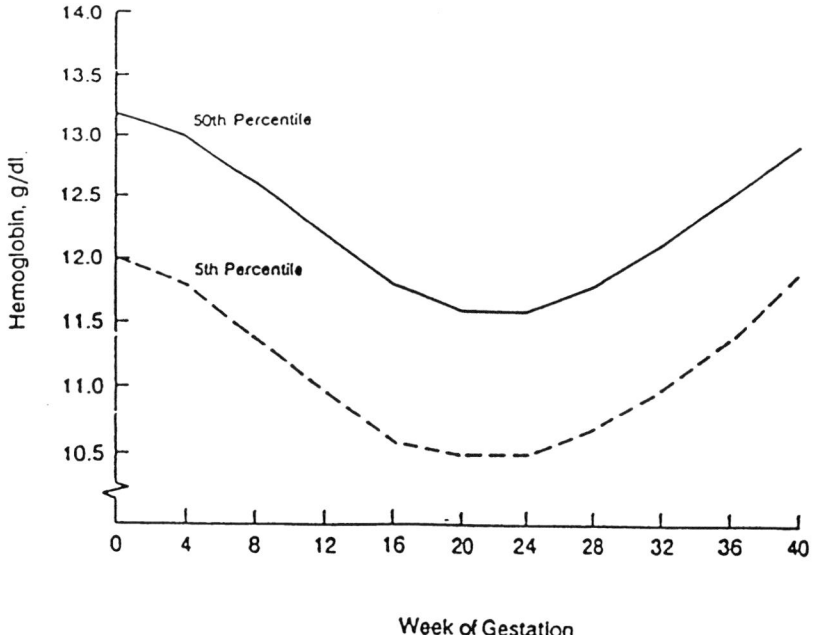

Week of Gestation

FIGURE B-16 Hemoglobin values during pregnancy. The hemoglobin concentration normally declines during the first half of pregnancy and rises during the second half. Values from 12 to 40 weeks of gestation are based on data from Svanberg et al. (1976), Sjöstedt et al. (1977), Puolakka et al. (1980), and Taylor et al. (1982). The baseline values (zero weeks) are based on LSRO (1984), and the 4- and 8-week values are extrapolated from all these data and from Clapp et al. (1988). SOURCE: CDC (1989).

TABLE B-4 Pregnancy Week-Specific Hemoglobin Cutoffs

Parameter	Cutoff by Week of Gestation[a]							
	12	16	20	24	28	32	36	40
Mean hemoglobin, g/dl	12.2	11.8	11.6	11.6	11.8	12.1	12.5	12.9
Fifth percentile hemoglobin values, g/dl	11.0	10.6	10.5	10.5	10.7	11.0	11.4	11.9
Equivalent fifth percentile hematocrit values, %	33.0	32.0	32.0	32.0	32.0	33.0	34.0	36.0

[a] For the sake of simplicity, hemoglobin cutoffs by trimester can be used as follows: 11.0 g/dl for the first and third trimesters, based on 12 and 32 weeks of gestation, respectively, and 10.5 g/dl, based on 24 weeks of gestation for the second trimester.

SOURCE: Based on pooled data from four European surveys of healthy women taking iron supplements (from CDC, 1989).

Figure B-16), largely because of a normal expansion in blood volume. From the end of the second trimester to term, the concentration of hemoglobin rises again.

Anemia is present only in those with hemoglobin concentrations that fall below the normal reference ranges for age, sex, and stage of pregnancy. Although iron deficiency is the most common cause of anemia, other causes include infection, hemoglobinopathies, and many other conditions. Although iron deficiency can result in anemia, high or excessive levels of iron intake do not increase the hemoglobin concentration beyond the normal range.

Iron Deficiency Anemia

Iron deficiency anemia refers to an anemia that is associated with additional laboratory evidence of iron depletion, such as a low serum ferritin concentration, transferrin saturation, or mean corpuscular volume (MCV) or an elevation in erythrocyte protoporphyrin or transferrin receptor levels. Table B-5 lists the cutoff values for these tests in children and adults.

TABLE B-5 Cutoff Values for Tests of Iron Status

Age, year	Serum Ferritin, µg/liter	Transferrin Saturation, %	Erythrocyte Protoporphyrin, µg/dl of red blood cells	MCV, fl
1–2	<10	<12	>80	<73
3–4	<10	<14	>75	<75
5–10	<10	<15	>70	<76
11–14	<10	<16	>70	<78
15–74	<12	<16	>70	<80

SOURCE: From LSRO (1984).

Serum ferritin concentration determination is the only laboratory test that allows the evaluation of iron reserves. A serum ferritin concentration of less than 10 µg/liter in children and less than 12 µg/liter in adults by itself indicates depleted iron stores (Table B-5). If an individual has already been found to be anemic, the likelihood of iron deficiency is greater than that in the general population. Under such circumstances, it may be appropriate to relax the cutoff value for the serum ferritin concentration. In combination with anemia, a value of less than 15 µg/liter indicates iron deficiency anemia.

Erythrocyte protoporphyrin accumulates in red blood cells when insufficient iron is available to form heme, the iron-containing portion of hemoglobin. It is most commonly measured on whole blood by a direct-readout instrument known as a hematofluorometer. Cutoff values are given in Table B-3. Erythrocyte protoporphyrin levels are elevated in individuals with iron deficiency or lead poisoning, as well as in those with infections or inflammatory conditions of more than 1 week in duration. In an otherwise healthy individual, anemia accompanied by an elevated protoporphyrin level is most commonly indicative of iron deficiency anemia.

Other laboratory tests used in the diagnosis of iron deficiency anemia include MCV, serum iron concentration and iron-binding capacity, and transferrin receptor concentration. MCV is one of the red blood cell indices that is provided by many laboratories when a hemoglobin concentration is ordered. A low MCV is most commonly associated with iron deficiency or thalassemia trait.

The ratio of serum iron to iron-binding capacity, expressed as a percentage (transferrin saturation), is decreased in individuals with iron deficiency. It is used less frequently than in the past because its colorimetric analysis requires freshly separated plasma and its reproducibility is relatively poor because of large biologic variations.

The determination of transferrin receptor concentration is a promising new test that should shortly become available for widespread use. The transferrin receptor concentration is elevated in individuals with iron deficiency but not in those with inflammatory disease, a useful feature, particularly when both conditions coexist (Ferguson et al., 1992). For nutritional survey purposes, the combination of transferrin receptor, serum ferritin, and hemoglobin concentrations is likely to provide an excellent depiction of iron status (Cook et al., 1993).

Iron Deficiency

The term iron deficiency can be applied to a lack of iron that is severe enough to impair the production of red blood cells but not necessarily to the extent that the hemoglobin concentration falls below the normal reference range. Iron deficiency can progress to iron deficiency anemia.

Iron Deficiency Without Anemia

Iron deficiency without anemia represents a relatively mild iron deficiency that is diagnosed on the basis of a combination of biochemical indicators of iron status but in which the hemoglobin concentration remains within the reference range. Unfortunately, no single indicator of iron status is diagnostic of iron deficiency. Cook et al. (1976) found that the prevalence of anemia among individuals with only one abnormal index of iron metabolism (low serum ferritin concentration, low serum iron concentration, low iron-binding capacity, or elevated erythrocyte protoporphyrin levels) was 11 percent, only slightly higher than the 8 percent in the entire population. In contrast, anemia was found in 28 percent of individuals with two abnormal values and 63 percent of those with three abnormal values. This finding and the analysis of data from the second National Health and Nutrition Examination Survey (NHANES II) suggested that for survey purposes, two or three abnormal biochemical indicators of iron status were more indicative of an iron deficiency of biologically significant severity than was a single indicator (LSRO, 1984). The term *impaired iron status* was applied to an abnormality in two or three of three biochemical tests.

Combinations of tests that have been used in large surveys include erythrocyte protoporphyrin and transferrin saturation determinations with either serum ferritin concentration or MCV determination (LSRO, 1984). The cost of doing multiple tests and the complexity of interpreting results for individuals make it difficult to detect this stage of iron deficiency except in nutrition surveys.

Rationale for Detecting Iron Deficiency by Screening for Anemia

Hemoglobin and hematocrit are most commonly used to screen for iron deficiency because they are easily analyzed and reflect the largest iron compartment in the body. Furthermore, physiologic impairment is associated almost entirely with iron deficiency anemia. However, many individuals with milder degrees of iron deficiency are missed by screening for anemia because of the overlap in values between normal and iron-deficient individuals. Hemoglobin and hematocrit values also vary with age, sex, and stage of pregnancy. This makes it important that clinicians use the appropriate cutoff values.

Use of a Second Laboratory Test

One approach to alleviating the problem of an overlap in hemoglobin and hematocrit values between normal and iron-deficient individuals is to use a second test to help ensure that individuals are accurately categorized and treated. If such tests are to be used in large populations, they must be relatively inexpensive and should preferably provide a result rapidly enough to allow initiation of treatment on the same visit. Tests that are widely used for this purpose are determination of erythrocyte protoporphyrin and serum ferritin concentrations. Transferrin receptor is the newest measure of iron status. Both transferrin receptor and erythrocyte protoporphyrin concentrations become elevated when there is a rate-limiting supply of iron to combine with erythrocyte protoporphyrin to form heme and eventually hemoglobin. They are therefore early indicators of physiologically significant iron deficiency. Studies to date indicate that the determination of transferrin receptor concentration will be particularly useful in the diagnosis of iron deficiency during pregnancy, because, like erythrocyte protoporphyrin, levels in iron-supplemented individuals remain stable throughout gestation (Carriaga et al., 1991; Cook et al., 1993), in contrast to the other measures of iron status.

Erythrocyte protoporphyrin levels are elevated in individuals with iron deficiency and lead poisoning, and are therefore used to screen infants and young children for both, particularly those who live in low-income urban areas, where the two conditions are most common. Test results can be obtained rapidly and at low cost. This laboratory measure has not been widely used to test pregnant subjects, but it deserves further study because it seems very promising (Schifman et al., 1987). Erythrocyte protoporphyrin levels remain stable throughout pregnancy in iron-supplemented women, but the levels rise in at least some unsupplemented women (Romslo et al., 1983).

Serum ferritin concentration is commonly determined in women, especially during pregnancy (IOM, 1990a). The serum ferritin concentration declines as iron stores decline. It is therefore valuable in predicting when iron deficiency is likely to develop during pregnancy in nonanemic women. Indeed, some advocate that pregnant women routinely be screened by determining their hemoglobin and serum ferritin concentrations (Hibbard, 1988). This option allows deferral of iron administration when both laboratory tests are normal. The results of Taylor et al. (1982) suggested that the serum ferritin concentration determination is less useful for this purpose in the last half of pregnancy because values decline to about 15 µg/liter even in iron-supplemented women. Less marked declines were also noted by Romslo et al. (1983). However, Puolakka et al. (1980) and Wallenburg and van Eijk (1984) found that mean serum ferritin concentrations did not fall below 45 and 47 µg/liter, respectively, in iron-supplemented women, compared with lows of 21 and 19 µg/liter, respectively, in the unsupplemented groups. There thus remains some degree of uncertainty about the usefulness of serum ferritin concentration determination in distinguishing iron-supplemented from unsupplemented and potentially iron-deficient individuals in the last half of pregnancy.

In nonpregnant women and children, a serum ferritin concentration of less than 12–15 µg/liter indicates that iron stores are very low, and a value in this range in combination with anemia provides strong evidence that the anemia is due to iron deficiency. Analysis of the serum ferritin concentration may be particularly useful for confirming that an anemia is due to iron deficiency, especially if it persists after iron treatment. This is especially applicable to blacks, among whom a slight depression in hemoglobin concentration may be normal (see below). Serum ferritin concentration analysis is also helpful for determining whether supplemental iron is necessary when it is poorly tolerated, despite adjustments in the iron supplementation regimen. If there is no anemia and if the serum ferritin concentration is not depressed, it is safe to delay iron supplementation until repeat analyses of serum ferritin indicate that iron stores have become very low. At present, the major disadvantage of the serum ferritin analysis is the delay in obtaining the results.

When routine screening is recommended for detecting iron deficiency among infants and women during their childbearing years, it is not cost-effective to use more than two or at the most three laboratory tests to distinguish iron-deficient from nondeficient individuals. The high cost of laboratory studies, the relatively poor sensitivity and specificity of hemoglobin and other iron status measures (Dallman and Reeves, 1984), and the rapid change from iron adequacy to iron deficiency over a few months argue against using a larger battery of tests.

Consequences of Iron Deficiency

Consequences of Iron Deficiency During Infancy and Childhood

Iron deficiency anemia can impair energy metabolism, temperature regulation, immune function, and work performance (Dallman, 1986). However, the consequence of greatest concern in infants is the impairment of mental and psychomotor development that is associated with even mild iron deficiency anemia. The studies of Walter et al. (1989) (Figure B-17), Lozoff et al. (1991), and Idjradinata and Pollitt (1993) indicate that significant deficits occur at 12 months of age with a hemoglobin concentration of less than 10.0 g/dl and may be present when the hemoglobin concentration is between 10.0 and 10.9 g/dl (<11.0 g/dl is the lower limit of the normal 95 percent reference range at this age). Iron treatment reversed the anemia, but in two of the studies (Lozoff et al., 1991; Walter et al., 1989), it was found that impaired cognitive function may remain evident 4 to 5 years later when the formerly anemic infants enter school. A different conclusion regarding the reversibility of mental and psychomotor delay in infants with iron deficiency anemia emerged from the recent study of Idjradinata and Pollitt (1993), in which a double-blind, iron versus placebo treatment trial provided strong evidence of complete recovery in response to iron treatment (Table B-6). The issue of reversibility remains the subject of intensive study. Earlier studies of Pollitt et al. (1989) also show that schoolchildren with iron deficiency anemia have poorer cognitive function, which is only partly improved by iron treatment. These results indicate that anticipation and prevention of iron deficiency anemia should have higher priorities than its detection. An emphasis on the detection of anemia alone may not ensure prevention of the harmful consequences of iron deficiency anemia.

Consequences of Iron Deficiency During Pregnancy

For many years, clinical studies of iron deficiency during pregnancy suggested that the fetus remained an effective parasite with respect to iron status, even though anemia developed in the mother (for reviews, see Hallberg, 1992, and IOM, 1990b). This conclusion was based on data showing that newborns of mothers with mild iron deficiency anemia at term were not anemic and had normal or only slightly diminished iron stores, as estimated on the basis of the serum ferritin concentration. During the past decade, this concept that the fetus is protected from maternal iron deficiency has been challenged by the observation that anemia, and more specifically, iron deficiency anemia, in early pregnancy is associated with prematurity and low birth weight in the newborn rather than with anemia, as one might have anticipated. In addition to concern about fetal development in relation to iron deficiency anemia, there are also probably disadvantages to the mother. Adults with iron deficiency anemia have increased lactic acid levels and tachycardia with exercise (see the review by Dallman, 1986). There is also a report indicating that adults with iron deficiency anemia have impaired attention spans and short-term memories (Groner et al., 1986).

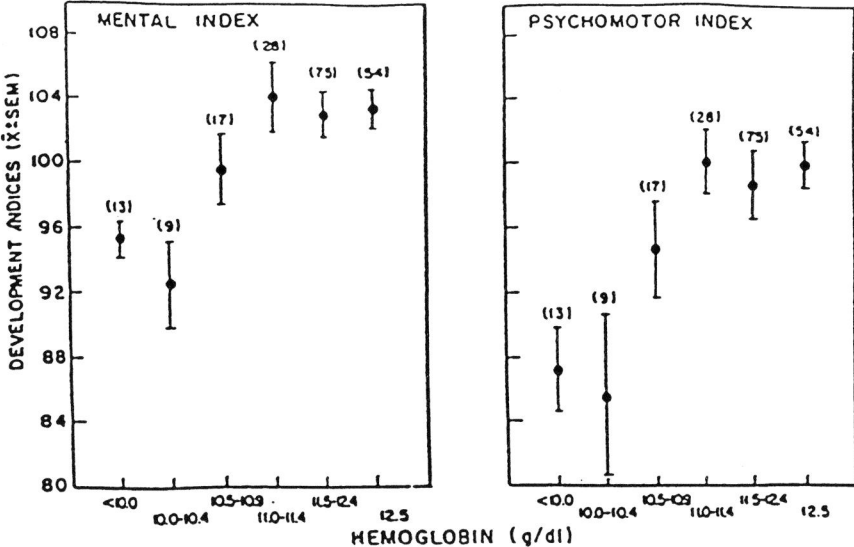

FIGURE B-17 Developmental delay in infants with iron deficiency anemia. Developmental indices (mean ± standard error of the mean) were lower in 12-month-old infants with iron deficiency anemia (hemoglobin concentration, <10.5 g/dl) than in nonanemic infants. SOURCE: From Walter et al. (1989).

Anemia and the Outcome of Pregnancy Large retrospective studies by Garn et al. (1981) and Murphy et al. (1986) showed that anemia early in pregnancy was associated with prematurity, low birth weight, and increased infant mortality. These findings were recently confirmed and expanded in a large survey by the Centers for Disease Control and Prevention (CDC) (Kim et al., 1992). Women who had hemoglobin concentrations of less than 10.0 g/dl in the first trimester had a significantly higher incidence of low-birth-weight babies (11 percent) compared with women with hemoglobin concentrations of 10.0 g/dl or greater (7 percent).

TABLE B-6 Developmental Delay in Infants with Iron Deficiency Anemia

Group and Time in Relation to Treatment	Hemoglobin, g/liter		Mental Score		Motor Score	
	Iron	Placebo	Iron	Placebo	Iron	Placebo
Iron deficiency anemia						
Before	96	98	89	92	86	92
After	129^a	107	108^a	93	112^a	98
Iron deficiency, no anemia						
Before	126	126	102	102	103	104
After	135^a	123	108	109	108	107
Iron sufficient						
Before	126	126	105	105	105	106
After	131	131	109	107	109	106

NOTE: Three groups of 12- to 18-month-old infants were enrolled in a double-blind, randomized iron versus placebo treatment trial for 4 months. Group 1 (n = 50) consisted of infants with iron deficiency anemia (hemoglobin concentration, <10.5 g/dl; transferrin saturation, ≤10 percent; serum ferritin concentration, <10 µg/liter). Group 2 (n = 29) consisted of infants with nonanemic iron deficiency (hemoglobin concentration, ≥12.0 g/dl; transferrin saturation, ≤10 percent; serum ferritin concentration, ≤12.0 µg/liter). Group 3 (n = 47) consisted of infants with iron sufficiency (hemoglobin concentration, ≥12.0 g/dl; transferrin saturation, >10 percent; serum ferritin concentration, ≥12.0 µg/liter). Abnormalities were reversed after 4 months of treatment.

$^a p<0.01$.

SOURCE: Idjradinata and Pollitt (1993).

Iron Deficiency Anemia and the Outcome of Pregnancy A recent study by Scholl and coworkers (1992) indicates that a poor birth outcome (low birth weight and prematurity) is linked more specifically to maternal iron deficiency anemia (anemia and a low serum ferritin concentration) early in pregnancy than to anemia per se (Table B-7). The statistical analysis adjusted for known confounders, including maternal age, parity, ethnicity, and stage of gestation at first blood draw. Thus, it seems likely that maternal iron deficiency anemia contributes to prematurity and low birth weight, which are the most common causes of infant morbidity and mortality. Iron deficiency anemia was also associated with poor maternal weight gain during gestation. These findings are in accord with those of another study suggesting a link between low serum ferritin concentration and preterm labor (Ulmer and Goepel, 1988).

What is still lacking is direct cause-and-effect evidence that prevention of iron deficiency anemia by iron supplementation decreases the risk of low birth weight and prematurity. Such a study, involving randomization of a large group to iron and placebo treatments, although highly desirable, may be difficult to mount in the United States, where iron supplementation is so widely recommended and practiced. There would also be ethical constraints in withholding iron treatment from individuals with anemia and low serum ferritin concentrations. Two expert committees of the Institute of Medicine (IOM, 1990a,1992) and one formed by the Life Sciences Research Office (LSRO, 1991) recently agreed on recommending routine low-dose iron (30 mg/day) for pregnant women on the basis of a careful evaluation of currently available evidence. As in the case of infants, the weight of evidence leads to the conclusion that anticipation and prevention of iron deficiency anemia deserve a high priority.

TABLE B-7 Associations of Anemia and Iron Deficiency Anemia with Inadequate Weight Gain and Pregnancy Outcome

	Anemia			
Outcome	Total	Iron Deficiency	Causes Other Than Iron Deficiency	No Anemia
Low birth weight				
Unadjusted, %	17.1	25.9	15.9	12.2
AOR[a]	1.55	3.10	1.34	1.00
95% Confidence interval	0.96–2.51	1.16–4.39	0.80–2.22	—
Preterm delivery				
Unadjusted, %	26.2	44.4	23.5	18.4
AOR[a]	1.30	2.66	1.16	1.00
95% Confidence interval	0.86–2.24	1.15–6.17	0.76–1.79	—
Small for gestational age				
Unadjusted, %	11.1	8.3	11.5	7.5
AOR[b]	1.66	1.24	1.67	1.00
95% Confidence interval	0.90–3.04	0.29–6.94	0.90–3.41	—
Inadequate weight gain				
Unadjusted, %	31.0	40.0	29.9	24.6
AOR[c]	1.62	2.67	1.51	1.00
95% Confidence interval	1.10–2.36	1.13–6.30	1.02–2.25	—

[a] AOR, adjusted odds ratio. Adjusted for maternal age, parity, ethnicity, prior low-birth-weight or preterm delivery, bleeding at entry, gestation at initial blood draw (entry), number of cigarettes smoked per day, and prepregnancy body mass index.
[b] Adjusted for maternal age, parity, prior low-birth-weight delivery, bleeding at entry, gestation at initial blood draw (entry), number of cigarettes smoked per day, and prepregnancy body mass index.
[c] Adjusted for maternal age, parity, ethnicity, bleeding at entry, gestation at initial blood draw (entry), and prepregnancy body mass index.

SOURCE: From Scholl et al. (1992).

EMERGING ISSUES AND FUTURE DIRECTIONS

Issues Involving the Possibility of Iron Excess

Iron is a micronutrient with a relatively narrow range of optimal levels of intake. Furthermore, individuals' iron requirements vary substantially by age and sex. These characteristics are relevant to the fortification of general-purpose foods with iron. Fortification of infant formula and cereal with iron has been a resounding success in reducing the prevalence of anemia in infants (Yip et al., 1987a,b), probably because these iron-fortified foods have been so well accepted by health professionals and parents.

Fortification of general-purpose cereal products for older children and adults has been more controversial (Crosby, 1986). Although children and women of childbearing age are the target population, men who are at little risk of iron deficiency actually consume the greatest quantities of the fortified products. The concern about iron excess pertains primarily to men and postmenopausal women and involves the following issues: disease caused by oxidative damage, increased risk of infection, and interaction of iron with other minerals. (See also Appendix C.)

Disease Caused by Oxidative Damage

Iron is a catalyst in free-radical reactions, such as lipid peroxidation, which can cause tissue damage. Iron-binding proteins in plasma and tissues offer protection against such damage by binding ionic iron, but there are reasons to suspect that this protection is incomplete (Cross et al., 1987; Weinberg, 1984). Specific conditions in which there may be an association of clinical disease with high iron stores include ischemic heart disease (Salonen et al., 1992). A high-iron diet is a disadvantage for individuals with hemochromatosis, who absorb excess iron, which increases the body's iron burden and is then believed to cause free-radical damage to tissues. There is also evidence that increased iron stores can be associated with an increased rate of growth of various forms of cancer (Weinberg, 1992).

Increased Risk of Infection

The iron-binding proteins transferrin and lactoferrin are believed to provide protection from infection by competitively binding the iron that invading bacteria require for their growth (Weinberg, 1984). This phenomenon has been called nutritional immunity and is the basis for concern that unneeded iron could predispose an individual to infection. There is a large body of experimental evidence that supports this concept. However, there is no convincing evidence that currently recommended iron fortification or treatment practices increase the risk of infection (Dallman, 1987).

Interaction of Iron with Other Minerals

Large doses of supplemental iron given to women (mean, 261 mg/day) resulted in a modest decline in plasma zinc levels (Hambidge et al., 1987). Another study of the relationship between iron and zinc or iron and copper indicated no such interaction (Sheldon et al., 1985). It remains uncertain whether the lower doses of iron that are currently recommended would increase the risk of zinc or copper deficiency. This question is relevant to the Institute of Medicine (1992) recommendation that if a therapeutic dose of iron (60–120 mg/day) is given, a multivitamin-mineral tablet containing 15 mg of zinc and 2 mg of copper given at a different time of the day should also be recommended. This would require two or three tablets per day and would result in poorer compliance than that with a simpler regimen of one tablet per day.

Race and Differences in Hemoglobin Concentration

The mean concentration of hemoglobin among groups of healthy blacks is consistently lower than that among a comparable, healthy white population of the same age and sex. This difference remains even when the populations have been screened to exclude those with iron deficiency and hemoglobinopathy and when the data are adjusted for socioeconomic differences. Indeed, the difference in hemoglobin concentration is similar in men and women, even though iron deficiency is a rarity among male adults. In NHANES II, this difference was 0.4 g/dl in children 3 to 4 years of age and 0.8 g/dl among both men and women between the ages of 20 and 44 years (LSRO, 1984). The whole hemoglobin distribution curve for blacks is shifted to the left of that for whites (Yip, 1989) (Figure B-18). The difference in hemoglobin concentration might be related to a very high prevalence of an α thalassemia gene among blacks (Beutler, 1988), but this has not been verified. Individuals with a single α thalassemia gene, unlike those with sickle trait and β thalassemia, are not detectable by hemoglobin electrophoresis, but only by laborious and costly techniques that are not clinically available. There does not appear to be any difference in hemoglobin values between whites and other racial groups, including Hispanics (Looker et al., 1989), East Asians (Dallman et al., 1978), Japanese (Uchida et al., 1988), and American Indians (Yip et al., 1984).

In general, the same hemoglobin criteria have been used for all races when screening women and children for anemia. This raises the problem that the percentage of black women and children who are erroneously suspected of having iron deficiency anemia is high enough to pose practical difficulties

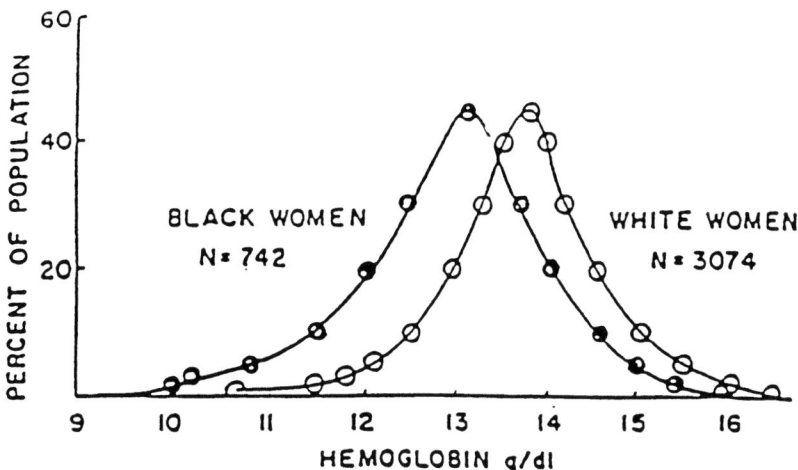

FIGURE B-18 Hemoglobin distributions among white and black women ages 18–44 years. The concentration of hemoglobin is lower among black women than among white women. The figure is based on data from NHANES I. SOURCE: From Yip (1989).

(Kim et al., 1992; Perry et al., 1992) (Figure B-19). Because blacks are more likely to be classified as anemic, they are more often subjected to unnecessary and expensive workups for anemia, needless concern about the possibility of disease, and the suspicion of poor compliance when there is no rise in hemoglobin concentration with iron therapy. The prevalence of anemia is substantially higher among pregnant black women than among those of other races. The difference between black and white or Hispanic women increases from about 8 percent in the first trimester to 15 to 20 percent in the third trimester (Figure B-19). It is uncertain to what extent the higher prevalence of "anemia" among black women, particularly late in pregnancy, is due to iron deficiency anemia. However, there is good evidence from NHANES II (LSRO, 1984) that black women have lower hemoglobin levels than white women even when their iron statuses are similar (Table B-8).

The problem of the specific criteria that should be used to diagnose anemia in blacks poses important health policy issues. Use of the same hemoglobin concentration criterion for women and children of all races is the simplest approach and recognizes the fact that not all blacks have low hemoglobin concentrations. However, many normal black individuals are incorrectly suspected of having iron deficiency anemia. This requires an awareness that the failure of a mild "anemia" in a black woman or child to respond to iron treatment is likely to indicate a normally low hemoglobin concentration and not necessarily a failure to take iron or an unusual anemia that requires further workup. The use of separate hemoglobin criteria for blacks could be seen as racially stigmatizing, but the advantage of fewer false-positive diagnoses is a strong argument for making an appropriate downward adjustment in hemoglobin and hematocrit cutoff values (Johnson-Spear and Yip, in press).

Absorption of Iron from Multivitamin-Mineral Supplements and Certain Foods

Less iron is absorbed from certain multivitamin-mineral supplements than from an equivalent amount of iron given alone. Calcium carbonate and magnesium oxide appear to be particularly inhibitory to iron absorption (Babior et al., 1985; Seligman et al., 1983). Seligman et al. (1983) found that iron absorption almost doubled when calcium as calcium carbonate was decreased from 350 to 250 mg and magnesium as magnesium oxide was decreased from 100 to 25 mg. The use of calcium supplements may also inhibit absorption of iron from foods under certain conditions (Hallberg et al., 1991). However, Galan et al. (1991) found no inhibition of iron absorption when calcium as milk or yogurt was added to a standard, meat-containing meal. These findings demonstrate the importance of additional research to determine the optimal ratios of nutrients in prenatal supplements and the relative merits of foods versus supplements as sources of certain nutrients. For the time being, if iron is given in the form of a prenatal supplement, it seems advisable to select products that contain about 60 mg of iron rather than use the dose of 30 mg that is recommended if iron is given alone. This would allow for an anticipated lower percentage of iron absorbed. It would also be best to select a formulation that contains no more than 250 mg of calcium.

Another area that needs further investigation is the availability of iron from certain foods, particularly breakfast cereals that contain iron and other micronutrients at the adult Recommended Dietary Allowance (RDA) equivalents. Specially formulated fortified foods targeted to women of childbearing age could be developed and might be of potential importance as vehicles for iron, folate, and possibly, calcium. With appropriate studies to verify the bioavailability of iron, such foods might be an attractive alternative to women for whom compliance in taking tablets is a problem.

Association of Neural Tube Defects with Folate Deficiency in Early Pregnancy: Implications for the Prevention of Iron Deficiency

The CDC recently recommended that all women of childbearing potential should consume 0.4 mg of folic acid per day for the purpose of reducing their risk of having a pregnancy affected with spina bifida or other neural tube defects (CDC, 1992). Currently in the United States, almost 2,500 infants are born with these defects each year. The recommendation was based largely on a recent investigation showing a reduced prevalence of first occurrence of neural tube defects in infants of women taking folate-containing supplements from

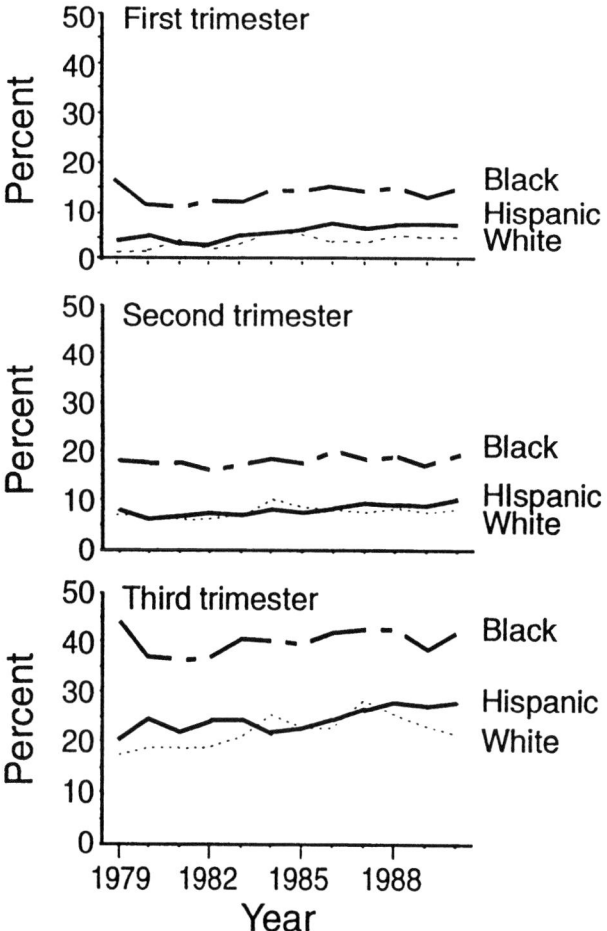

FIGURE B-19 Antepartum anemia, by racial or ethnic group and trimester, determined as part of the Pregnancy Nutrition Surveillance System, United States, 1979–1990. The prevalence of anemia increases with the progression of pregnancy. There has been no decrease in the prevalence of anemia during the period monitored, a decade during which there was a marked diminution of anemia among infants and preschool children. The consistently higher prevalence of anemia among blacks than among Hispanics or whites (about 8 percent in the first trimester, 10 percent in the second trimester, and 15 to 20 percent in the third trimester) is partly due to the lower hemoglobin concentrations in blacks, even those with normal iron status. SOURCE: From Kim et al. (1992).

TABLE B-8 Prevalence of Anemia and Iron Deficiency Among White and Black Women from 20 to 44 Years of Age

	Percent	
Condition	White	Black
Anemia	9.0	25
Iron deficiency	5.0 ± 0.6^a	5.7 ± 0.9

NOTE: Anemia was defined as a hemoglobin concentration of <12.0 g/dl. Individuals were designated as having iron deficiency when results of two or three tests (MCV, transferrin saturation, and erythrocyte protoporphyrin) were abnormal. Although anemia was much more common among blacks than among whites, the prevalence of iron deficiency was similar.

^{a} Values are means ± standard errors of the means.

SOURCE: LSRO (1984).

at least 1 month before conception to the date of the second missed menstrual period or later (Czeizel and Dudas, 1992). Several earlier studies indicated that the prevalence of recurrent neural tube defects could be decreased by folate supplementation.

The relevance of the CDC recommendation to iron supplementation is that many more women of childbearing age will be taking folate in the form of a multivitamin-mineral preparation that also contains iron before they are pregnant and during early pregnancy. The recent studies associating iron deficiency anemia or anemia in early pregnancy with low birth weight will also foster increased and earlier use of iron supplements.

Between 1976 and 1980, 38 percent of women between the ages of 18 and 50 reported taking a vitamin supplement, a mineral supplement, or both (Laplan et al., 1986). In the more recent 1987 Health Interview Survey, 27 percent of women reported daily supplement use, and for 20 percent this was a multivitamin-mineral supplement (Subar and Block, 1990). The prospects of increasing the use of vitamin-mineral supplements as a vehicle for iron supplementation make it imperative that there be more investigation of the availability of iron from such preparations, as suggested above. Since folate-fortified foods are being considered as a means of supplying extra folate to women of childbearing age, there is also the need to investigate the prospects for developing special fortified foods targeted to young women. Such food could respond to concerns not only about folate deficiency but also about iron deficiency, osteoporosis, and other problems primarily involving this group.

Iron Supplements Often Are Not Taken Regularly

Recommendations to use iron supplements have little prospect for success unless they are likely to result in reasonably good compliance. Unfortunately, compliance can be surprisingly inconsistent even for relatively simple drug regimens used for life-threatening conditions like epilepsy, diabetes, hypertension, and organ transplantation (Haynes et al., 1979). The problem is likely to be even greater when the individual has no obvious illness. Bonnar et al. (1969) monitored compliance by measuring iron levels in the stools of pregnant women who were advised to take ferrous fumarate at a dose of 65 mg of iron twice a day. About one-third failed to take iron, and this proportion was even greater among those who were initially anemic. The poor compliance could not be attributed to gastrointestinal side effects, since these were extremely rare.

The side effects of iron therapy would contribute to poor compliance, but their prevalence has been most thoroughly investigated in double-blind studies with doses higher than those recommended in this report. At a dose of 65 mg of iron as ferrous sulfate taken three times a day, about 25 percent of subjects had side effects, whereas 13 percent of those receiving a placebo experienced side effects (Hallberg et al., 1967; Sölvell, 1970). With a doubling of the dose, the prevalence of side effects increased to 40 percent. There is little information about side effects at lower doses, but evidence of dose dependency and the study of Bonnar et al. (1969) cited above make it unlikely that doses of 30 mg of iron once a day or 60 mg twice a day would be a major deterrent to compliance. Nevertheless, it would be helpful to have more information on side effects at these lower doses.

Improving Compliance

What can be done to improve compliance? Compliance can be improved by using strong motivational techniques and frequent follow-up. Under ordinary circumstances, however, especially in busy and understaffed clinics, it seems likely that poor compliance is frequently responsible for a failure to treat or prevent iron deficiency anemia. The most effective single approach is to simplify the treatment regimen. Compliance was found to be substantially better with once-a-day iron therapy than with three-times-a-day medication (Porter, 1969) (Figure B-20). A similar result was obtained with long-term treatment for epilepsy (Cramer et al., 1989). Compliance averaged 87 percent with once-daily treatment, 81 percent with twice-daily treatment, 77 percent with three-times-daily treatment, and 39 percent with four-times-daily treatment. It would clearly be desirable to fill all supplement needs whenever possible with a single tablet taken once a day.

There are additional measures that are likely to be helpful in improving compliance (Haynes, 1979) (Table B-9). It is important that the health care provider explain why the medication will benefit the patient or her child. Medication is most likely to be taken if the health care provider provides written or printed instructions. Taking of medication should be linked to an already established daily routine like toothbrushing. On revisits to an office or clinic, it is important for the health care provider to reinforce the use of the supplement by asking about it and stressing its importance. Even so, compliance is likely to drop off between visits. A group of epileptic patients averaged 88 percent compliance before and 86 percent after a clinic visit, but this dropped to 67 percent compliance a month later (Cramer et al., 1990).

Iron Deficiency Increases the Risk of Lead Toxicity

Iron deficiency is associated with increased levels of lead in the blood of preschool children (Clark et al., 1988). The basis for this association is probably the shared absorptive mechanism for the two metals. Lead absorption is increased in individuals with iron deficiency. Since lead toxicity impairs cognitive function (as does iron deficiency), this risk is another justification for preventing iron deficiency.

As mentioned above, iron-fortified foods have been remarkably effective in reducing the prevalence of iron deficiency anemia among infants and preschool children, thereby decreasing the vulnerability to lead poisoning. Environmental exposure to lead has decreased since leaded gasoline has been removed from the market (Annest et al., 1983); removal of additional lead from the environment will be much more costly. At present, prevention of iron deficiency anemia is probably the most cost-effective way of further decreasing the risk of lead poisoning.

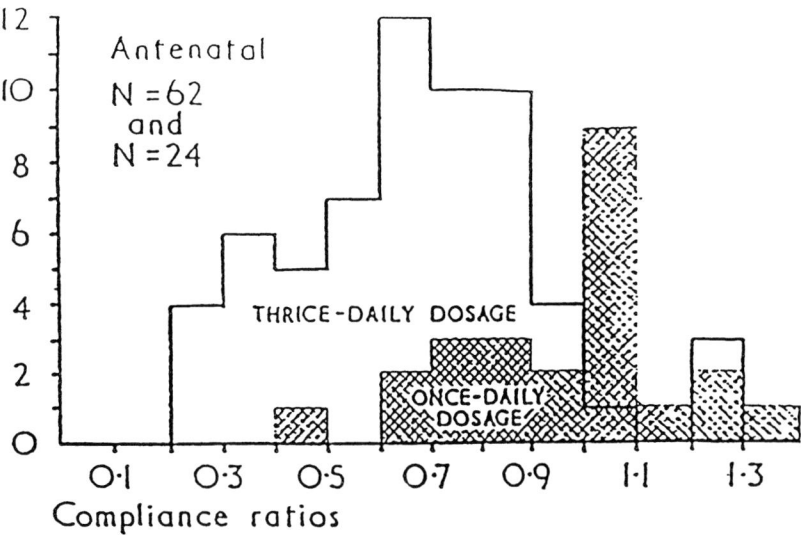

FIGURE B-20 Distribution of compliance ratios for antenatal patients on thrice- daily and once-daily iron preparations (compliance ratio is the number of tablets actually taken by the patient divided by the number of tablets that should have been taken). SOURCE: Based on Porter (1969).

TABLE B-9 Methods for Improving Compliance

1. Explain how the medication will benefit the patient or her child.
2. Provide written instructions.
3. Link taking of medication to an established daily routine, like toothbrushing.
4. Schedule follow-up visits and telephone "no-shows."
5. Reinforce use of supplement by asking about it and stressing its importance.

IRON DEFICIENCY ANEMIA IN INFANTS AND CHILDREN: PREVALENCE AND RECENT RECOMMENDATIONS

Magnitude of the Problem

Iron deficiency is common among infants and children from about 6 months to 3 years of age, but its prevalence has been declining over the past two decades. The most recent information on the prevalence of iron deficiency in the U.S. population as a whole, which was collected between 1976 and 1980, is from NHANES II. NHANES III is now in progress and should soon provide more up-to-date information. In NHANES II, the prevalence of iron deficiency was about 9 percent in infants aged 1 to 2 years, which was determined by using the same laboratory criteria (on the basis of MCV, transferrin saturation, and erythrocyte protoporphyrin) that yielded a prevalence of 5 percent among women during their childbearing years. Since then, the prevalence of iron deficiency anemia in infants and preschool children has been declining drastically on the basis of the prevalence of anemia in clinics that participate in the U.S. Department of Agriculture's Supplemental Food Program for Women, Infants, and Children (WIC) (Yip et al., 1987b) (Figure B-21) and in private practice settings (Yip et al., 1987a) (Figure B-22). In WIC clinics, the prevalence of anemia declined in a linear fashion, from 7 percent in children born in 1973 to 3 percent in those born in 1984. Stricter criteria for anemia than those commonly used in a clinical setting (hemoglobin, <10.3 g/dl; hematocrit, <31 percent) were applied to evaluate trends more accurately because of evidence that reporting of the measurements was influenced by the enrollment requirements for WIC. The actual values are apt to underestimate the prevalence of anemia by more widely used clinical criteria (AAP, CON, 1993; Dallman and Siimes, 1979). In a middle-class population, the prevalence of anemia on the basis of the widely used cutoff of a hematocrit level of less than 33 percent between the ages of 9 and 23 months declined from 7 percent between 1969 and 1973 to less than 3 percent between 1982 and 1986 (Figure B-22). The latter is close to the statistical baseline level for a normal population, suggesting that there remains little or no iron deficiency anemia in this study population. These striking improvements can be attributed to changes in infant feeding practices that took place during this period: later introduction of cow's milk and greater use of iron-fortified formula (Fomon, 1987). The incorporation of iron-fortified formula in the WIC food package for infants is believed to have played a major role in the decline of anemia among infants from lower socioeconomic groups.

In screening for anemia, mild infection has come to be recognized as an important confounding factor. Young children commonly have mild upper respiratory infections, gastroenteritis, or otitis media on health care visits. In one study, the prevalence of anemia between 1982 and 1986 in children with illnesses averaged about 7 percent compared with 3 percent in those from the same population who were entirely well (Yip, 1989) (Figure B-23). Even a history of a recent infection or evidence of an inflammatory process (on the basis of erythrocyte sedimentation rate) is associated with a much higher prevalence of anemia and low-normal hemoglobin values (Figure B-24). These findings emphasize the importance of testing for anemia to screen for iron deficiency only when an individual is and has recently been free of infection.

Preterm Infants

Studies comparing the concentration of hemoglobin and other iron status measures in iron-supplemented and unsupplemented infants show that those with a birth weight of less than 2,000 g are at very high risk of developing iron deficiency anemia after 2 months of age unless they receive an iron supplement, iron-fortified formula, or both (Lundström et al., 1977) (Figure B-11).

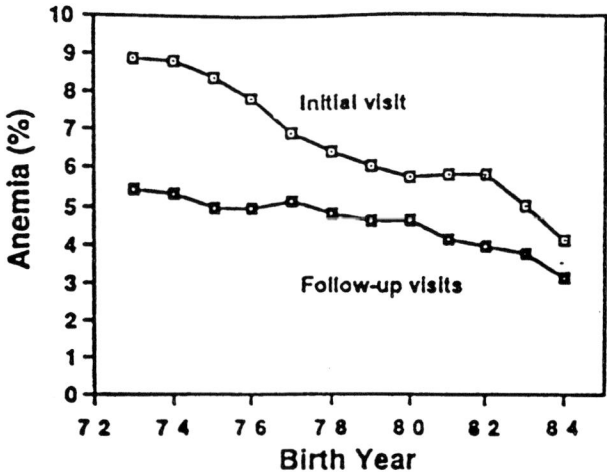

FIGURE B-21 Prevalence of anemia among infants and children in WIC clinics. The lower prevalence in children already in the WIC program is associated with the use of iron-fortified infant formula and other foods intended to improve iron status. SOURCE: Comparison of anemia trends of non-WIC and WIC children is based on data from the CDC Pediatric Nutrition Surveillance System, 1976–1985, from Yip et al. (1987b).

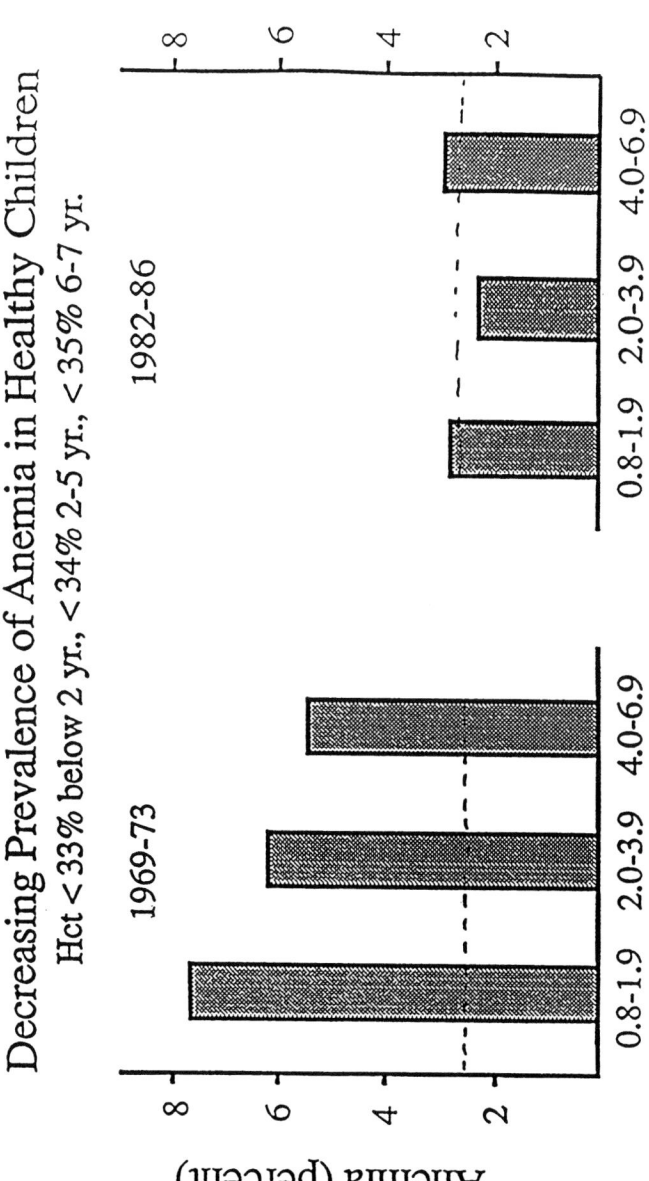

FIGURE B-22 Prevalence of anemia among a group of middle-class U.S. children from 0.8 to 6.9 years of age. Anemia has become rare among middle-class children. Between 1969 and 1981, there was a decline in the prevalence of anemia with increasing age. Between 1982 and 1986, the prevalence of anemia in all age ranges fell close to the theoretical minimum of 2.5 percent (horizontal dashed line). Hematocrit cutoff values for anemia are <33 percent for those younger than 2 years of age, <34 percent for those from 2 to 5 years of age, and <35 percent for those from 6 to 7 years of age. SOURCE: From Yip et al. (1987a).

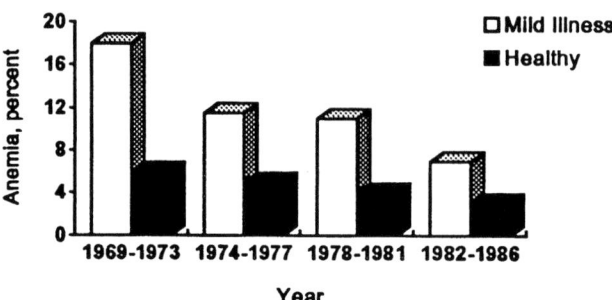

FIGURE B-23 Comparison of the prevalence of anemia among healthy children and those with a mild illness over four time periods on the basis of data from a middle-class pediatric practice. The prevalence of anemia in children with a mild infection is much higher than the prevalence of anemia in healthy children. Both have been declining over the past two decades. SOURCE: Adapted from Yip et al. (1987a).

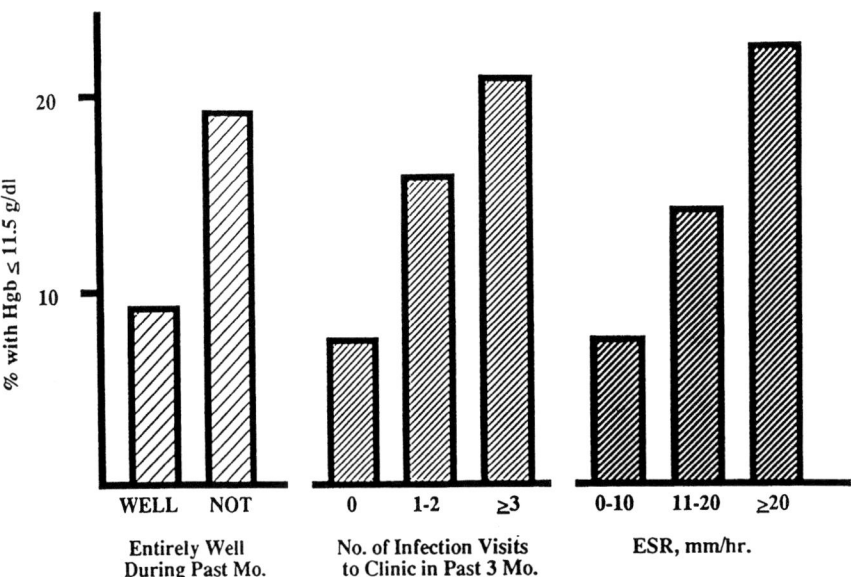

FIGURE B-24 Effect of recent infection or inflammatory process on anemia and hemoglobin value. Anemia and low to normal hemoglobin concentration are more common among healthy 1-year-old infants with a history of recent mild infection than among those who have been entirely well. ESR is erythrocyte sedimentation rate. SOURCE: From Reeves et al. (1984).

Preschool Children, School-Age Children, and Adolescents

After age 3 years, the risk of iron deficiency anemia is less (Yip et al., 1987a,b) (Figure B-22). When children are served meals in day care or at schools, there is an opportunity to provide foods that meet nutrition guidelines for iron and other nutrients. In adolescence, it becomes more difficult to meet the increasing iron needs (Hallberg et al., in press; Widholm et al., 1967) because meals are often eaten with less regularity and snack foods may substitute for what was previously a more varied diet. It is also a challenge to screen teenagers for anemia because it is uncommon for them to be seen for annual health maintenance checkups as recently recommended by the American Medical Association Panel on Adolescent Health (AMA, 1992).

Review of Earlier Guidelines for Prevention and Treatment

Committee on Nutrition, American Academy of Pediatrics

The Committee on Nutrition (CON) of the American Academy of Pediatrics (AAP) has issued a number of statements on iron nutrition and iron metabolism since 1969. For the most part, the recommendations have remained the same. The changes during that period have involved mainly the duration for which iron-fortified formula was to be used and the age before which cow's milk should not be started in the diets of infants. The recommendations for term and preterm infants that apply currently can be summarized as follows.

Term Infants On the basis of an extensive review of iron balance in infancy, the recommended total iron intake for term infants is 1 mg/kg/day to a maximum of 15 mg/kg/day (AAP, CON, 1969). All formula-fed infants should receive an iron-fortified formula (AAP, CON, 1989) until 12 months of age. Iron-fortified formula supplies ample iron to meet the iron requirements of infants. Breastfed infants should be weaned to an iron-fortified formula rather than to cow's milk if they are weaned before 12 months of age. Cow's milk and low-iron formulas should not be fed during the first 12 months of life (AAP, CON, 1992). Iron-fortified infant cereal is recommended when infants start solid foods (AAP, CON, 1969, 1976).

Preterm Infants The recommended total iron intake for preterm infants is 2 to 3 mg/kg/day to a maximum of 15 mg/kg/day (AAP, CON, 1969, 1985). Iron supplementation for low-birth-weight infants should start when the infant reaches a body weight of about 2,000 g or goes home. Infants fed human milk should receive 2 to 3 mg of elemental iron (per kg/day) as ferrous sulfate drops. If oral iron supplements are started earlier, at 2 weeks or when enteral feedings are tolerated, a dose of 2 to 3 mg/kg/day as well as a vitamin E supplement should be given. Formulas with iron usually contain sufficient iron so that no additional iron supplement is needed. Breastfed infants should be weaned to an iron-fortified formula rather than to cow's milk if they are weaned before 12 months of age. Cow's milk and low-iron formulas should not be fed during the first 12 months (AAP, CON, 1992). Iron-fortified infant cereal is recommended when infants start solid foods (AAP, CON, 1967, 1976).

Canadian Paediatric Society

Breastfed infants should be fed iron-fortified cereal (Canadian Paediatric Society, Nutrition Committee, 1991). Iron-fortified formula should be fed to infants who are not breastfed. Cow's milk should not be started until after 9 to 12 months of age. Iron supplements for low-birth-weight infants should start by 8 weeks of age and should be maintained until 12 months of age.

Recommended Dietary Allowances, 10th Edition

Infants to Age 3 Years For infants from birth to age 3 years, 1 mg of iron per kg/day was recommended for those who are not breastfed, but it was noted that satisfactory levels of hemoglobin could be maintained without extra iron from birth to age 3 months. The RDA for iron for those aged 6 months to 3 years was set at 10 mg/day. For low-birth-weight infants with birth weights of from 1,000 to 2,500 g, 2 mg/kg/day was recommended starting no later than 2 months of age. The maximum iron intake was set at 15 mg/day for term and low-birth-weight infants (NRC, 1989).

Children Ages 3 Years and Older For children, the RDA for iron was set at 10 mg/day, with an increase at age 10 years to 12 mg/day for males and 15 mg/day for females (NRC, 1989).

IRON DEFICIENCY IN WOMEN OF CHILDBEARING POTENTIAL: PREVALENCE AND RECENT RECOMMENDATIONS

Magnitude of the Problem

In contrast to children in whom inadequate iron intake is usually responsible for iron deficiency, excessive iron losses via menstrual blood and pregnancy play major roles among women of childbearing age. Also in contrast to children, there is no evidence that the prevalence of iron deficiency among women of childbearing age has declined substantially during the past two decades.

NHANES II (1976–1980)

In this large national survey, about 5–10 percent of women between the ages of 20 and 44 years in the United States were iron deficient on the basis of two or three abnormal values for indicators of iron status (Expert Scientific Working Group, 1985; LSRO, 1984). Five percent were iron deficient on the basis of an abnormal MCV, transferrin saturation, and erythrocyte protoporphyrin values; and 10 percent were iron deficient on the basis of abnormal serum ferritin, transferrin saturation, and/or erythrocyte protoporphyrin values. In contrast, less than 1 percent of men between the ages of 20 and 44 years were iron deficient by these criteria.

Females between the ages of 15 and 19 years had a prevalence of iron deficiency similar to that for women aged 20 to 44 years. The prevalence of iron deficiency among women between 20 and 44 years of age was greater with poverty, brief education, and high parity (LSRO, 1984) (Table B-10). There is no information on the prevalence of iron deficiency among a national sample of pregnant women.

About 8 percent of white women were anemic (hemoglobin concentration, <12.0 g/dl), and about 3 percent had iron deficiency anemia (anemia plus two or three abnormal hemoglobin values). These analyses were reported for whites only because many more blacks would be identified as anemic, despite having normal iron status (as discussed above; see Table B-8).

Pregnancy Nutrition Surveillance System—United States, 1979–1990

This CDC Surveillance System monitored nutritional risk factors among low-income pregnant women participating in public health programs. A recent

TABLE B-10 Risk Factors for Iron Deficiency

Risk Factor	Percent with Iron Deficiency
Economic status	
Above poverty level	5.1 ± 0.5 *
Below poverty level	7.8 ± 1.5 *
Education	
None/elementary school	13.4 ± 2.8 ** +
High school	5.4 ± 0.6 **
College	4.2 ± 0.6 +
Parity	
0	3.1 ± 0.5
1–2	3.8 ± 0.8
3–4	9.4 ± 1.1 ++
>5	11.1 ± 2.1 ++

NOTE: Iron deficiency is defined as two or three abnormal values for the following tests: MCV, transferrin saturation, and erythrocyte protoporphyrin. Prevalence of iron deficiency is shown for women between 20 and 44 years of age. Significance: *, $p < 0.10$; **, $p < 0.05$; +, $p < 0.01$; ++, $p < 0.005$ (in both other groups).

SOURCE: LSRO (1984).

report based on this survey (Kim et al., 1992) showed a prevalence of anemia that was high and that increased during the course of pregnancy. In 1990, for example, about 5, 8, and 25 percent of white and Hispanic women were anemic in the first, second, and third trimesters, respectively, indicating a worsening of iron status during the progression of pregnancy as iron needs increase (Figure B-19). Most discouraging was the finding that the prevalence of anemia has remained stable or has increased slightly since 1979 (Figure B-19), a period during which there has been a marked decline in anemia among infants and preschool-age children served by the same clinics (Figure B-21). These findings indicate a need for new approaches to the prevention of anemia and iron deficiency among low-income, pregnant women.

Black women had a disproportionately high prevalence of anemia compared with white and Hispanic women. The discrepancy increases progressively from the first to the second and third trimesters. The high prevalence is partly related to the lower hemoglobin concentrations in blacks, even when iron status is normal. The extent to which iron deficiency also plays a role in the higher prevalence of anemia among blacks, particularly in the second and third trimesters, remains uncertain. The findings do show that the interpretation of anemia among pregnant black women requires special attention to minimize the false diagnosis of anemia and iron deficiency.

Clinical Trials in Iron-Supplemented versus Unsupplemented Pregnant Women

Several carefully performed studies in which iron-supplemented and unsupplemented women were followed at monthly intervals during pregnancy were recently summarized (Table B-4). In all cases, the women studied were not anemic on their first prenatal visit. However, the mean hemoglobin concentration became lower in unsupplemented than in iron-supplemented women after about 24 weeks of gestation, and the difference, as illustrated by one of these studies (Taylor et al., 1982), continued to increase with the progression of pregnancy (Figure B-25). The increasing prevalence of anemia during the course of pregnancy is in accord with the survey data described above for the Pregnancy Nutrition Surveillance System.

Review of Current Guidelines

Committee on Professional Standards, American College of Obstetricians and Gynecologists

As early in pregnancy as possible, the clinician should determine the hemoglobin concentration or hematocrit (a venipuncture will be required for the additional laboratory tests that are recommended). The hemoglobin or hematocrit analysis should be repeated again early in the third trimester (ACOG, 1989).

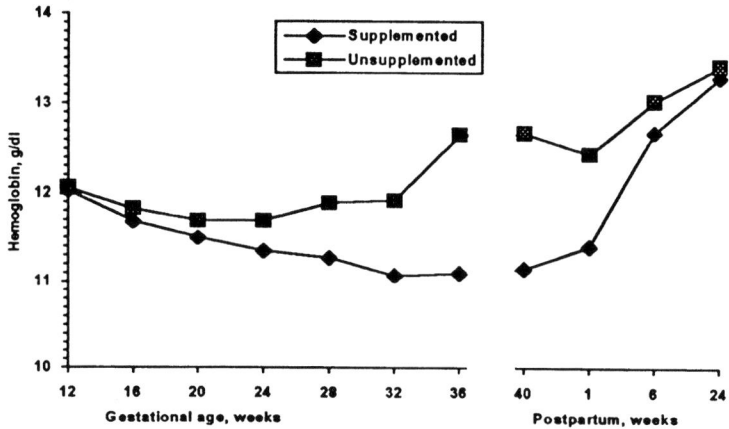

FIGURE B-25 Hemoglobin concentration during gestation and postpartum in women receiving an iron supplement and women not supplemented with iron. The unsupplemented group had a lower mean hemoglobin concentration after about 24 weeks of gestation, and differences became more marked during the progression of pregnancy. After delivery, differences in hemoglobin concentration disappear as the blood volume decreases. SOURCE: Data from Taylor et al. (1982).

Nutritional status should be evaluated on the initial visit and should be monitored on subsequent visits throughout the pregnancy. If iron, folate, and certain other vitamin needs are not met by the diet, the clinician should recommend a vitamin-mineral supplement that supplies the RDAs for pregnant women.

The recommended frequency of visits is every 4 weeks for the first 28 weeks of gestation, every 2 to 3 weeks until 36 weeks of gestation, and weekly thereafter.

Institute of Medicine: Nutrition During Pregnancy *and* Nutrition During Pregnancy and Lactation: An Implementation Guide

Nutrition During Pregnancy (IOM, 1990a) included a chapter on iron nutrition during pregnancy with a review of the literature (IOM, 1990b). That review concluded with the recommendations outlined below. The *Implementation Guide*, which was published 2 years later (IOM, 1992), was prepared as a briefer user manual for improving nutrition during pregnancy and lactation. It included more specific clinical information, which is also summarized below.

Eat a well-balanced diet (*Dietary Guidelines for Americans*, DHHS/USDA, 1991) that contains enhancers of iron absorption (ascorbic acid, meat).

Routinely determine the hemoglobin concentration or hematocrit on the first prenatal visit to detect preexisting anemia. A hemoglobin level of less than 11.0 g/dl during the first or third trimesters or less than 10.5 g/dl during the second trimester is defined as anemia.

Nonanemic women should routinely take about 30 mg of ferrous iron beginning at about the 12th week of gestation. Take the iron between meals and with water or juice, but not with milk, tea, or coffee. The rationale for the 30-mg dose is that it is the lowest for which there is strong evidence of effectiveness (Chanarin and Rothman, 1971) (Figure B-26). Such low doses can be relatively effective because the percentage of iron absorbed decreases as the dose increases. Thus, a more than sixfold increase in dose from 18 to 120 mg scarcely doubles the amount of iron absorbed (B-Figure 27) (Hahn et al., 1951). It was considered equally important to select a low dose to avoid the relatively high prevalence of side effects seen with the commonly employed regimens of 180 mg/day. The lower dose could be given as a single tablet once a day, favoring compliance.

Anemia accompanied by a serum ferritin concentration of less than 12 µg/liter can be presumed to be iron deficiency anemia and requires treatment with 60 to 120 mg of ferrous iron daily (no more than about 60 mg per dose). Hemoglobin or hematocrit should be checked again after about 1 month. When the hemoglobin or hematocrit becomes normal for the stage of gestation, the dose can be decreased to 30 mg/day. A persistent anemia requires questions about compliance or further laboratory studies to consider other causes of anemia.

Nutrition During Pregnancy and Lactation: An Implementation Guide (IOM, 1992) A preconception or interconception visit should include a screening for anemia with the determination of hemoglobin concentration or hematocrit. A hemoglobin concentration of less than 12.0 g/dl was defined as anemia (Table B-4). Corrections for smoking and residence at high altitude were provided (Table B-11). The determination of serum ferritin should be considered in women with anemia. A serum ferritin concentration of less than 20 µg/liter with anemia indicates iron deficiency as the cause of anemia.

The use of a folate-containing supplement to help prevent recurrent neural tube defects was mentioned as relevant to iron supplementation, since it offers the possibility of using a vitamin-mineral supplement containing both iron and folate.

Prenatal multivitamin-mineral supplements were recommended for women identified to be at high nutritional risk. Table B-12 shows the suggested composition of such supplements.

A brief dietary history was recommended on this and the first prenatal visit. Dietary advice based on *Dietary Guidelines for Americans* was also suggested for both visits (DHHS/USDA, 1991).

The first prenatal visit includes screening for anemia. Anemia was defined as a hemoglobin concentration of less than 11.0 g/dl in the first or third

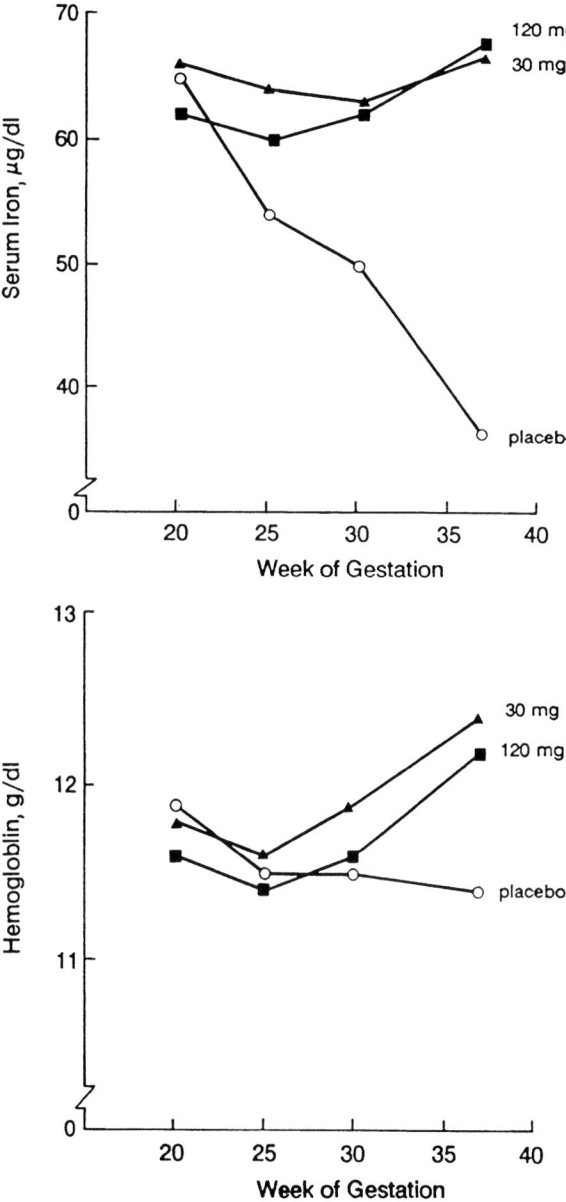

FIGURE B-26 Serum iron and hemoglobin levels in groups of 46 to 49 randomly assigned women receiving either a placebo or various doses of elemental iron as ferrous fumarate given orally on a daily basis. Data from groups receiving 60-mg oral doses of iron or 1 g of iron given parenterally and then 60-mg oral doses of iron per day are not shown but are similar to those of the iron-supplemented groups shown in the figure. Note that daily doses of 30 and 120 mg were similarly effective in preventing anemia. SOURCE: From IOM (1990a), based on Chanarin and Rothman (1971).

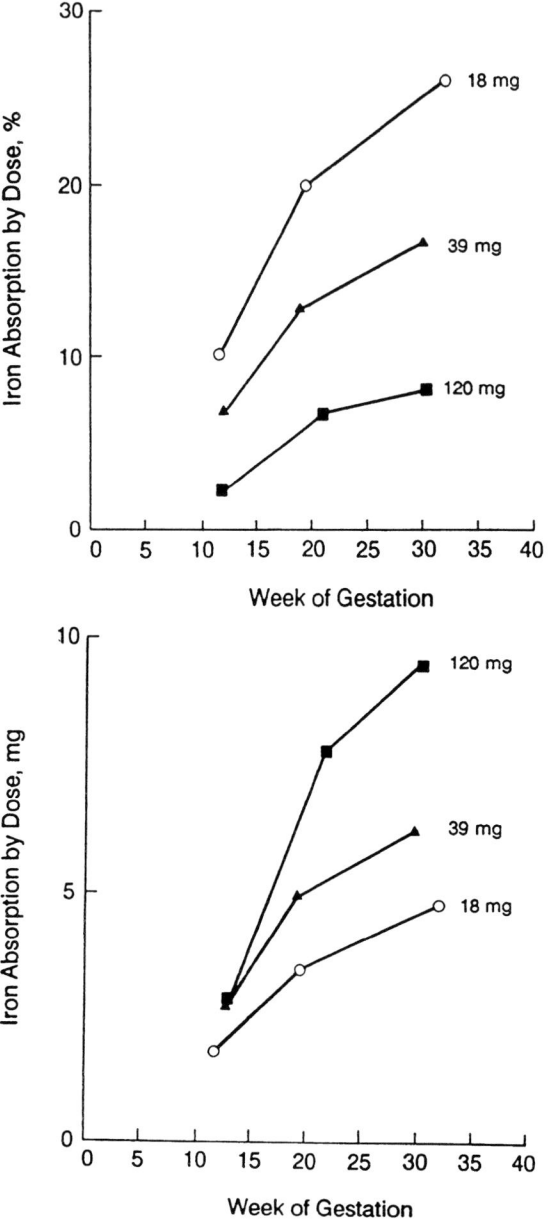

FIGURE B-27 Absorption of iron (as a percentage of the dose above and in milligrams below) in relation to dose and stage of pregnancy, based on data from Hahn et al. (1951). Iron absorption increased during the progression of pregnancy. At any stage of pregnancy, the percentage of iron absorbed decreases as the dose of iron increases. At about 30 weeks of gestation, a more than sixfold increase in dose from 18 to 120 mg of iron only doubles the amount of iron absorbed. SOURCE: IOM (1990a).

TABLE B-11 Cutoff Values for Anemia in Women of Childbearing Age

Group	Hemoglobin (g/dl)[a]	Hematocrit (%)[a]
Nonpregnant women		
Nonsmokers	12.0	36
10–20 cigarettes/day	12.3	37
20–40 cigarettes/day	12.5	37.5
Pregnant women		
Nonsmokers		
First trimester	11.0	33
Second trimester	10.5	32
Third trimester	11.0	33
10–20 cigarettes/day		
First trimester	11.3	34
Second trimester	10.8	33
Third trimester	11.3	34
21–40 cigarettes/day		
First trimester	11.5	34.5
Second trimester	11.0	33.5
Third trimester	11.5	34.5

[a] For altitudes of about 5,000 ft. (i.e., Denver, Salt Lake City), add 0.5 g/dl to the hemoglobin cutoff or 1.5 percent to the hematocrit cutoff.

SOURCES: IOM (1992) and CDC (1989).

TABLE B-12 Suggested Composition (approximate) of Prenatal Daily Vitamin-Mineral Supplements for Use by Women Identified To Be At High Nutritional Risk[a]

Nutrient	Amount
Iron	30–60 mg
Zinc	15 mg
Copper	2 mg
Calcium[b]	250 mg
Vitamin D	10 µg (400 IU)
Vitamin C	50 mg
Vitamin B_6	2 mg
Folate	300 µg
Vitamin B_{12}	2 µg

[a] If vitamin A is included, β-carotene is preferred over retinol, to reduce the risk of toxicity or other adverse reactions.

[b] Since calcium and magnesium may interfere with iron absorption, upper limits of 250 and 23 mg per dose, respectively, are recommended as a part of vitamin-mineral supplements. Some calcium supplements provide less than the recommended 600 mg of elemental calcium per tablet. It is advisable to take supplements containing calcium alone (e.g., calcium carbonate) with meals to promote absorption of the calcium.

SOURCE: Adapted from IOM (1992).

trimester and less than 10.5 g/dl in the second trimester. The routine use of ferrous iron at a dose of about 30 mg/day was recommended for nonanemic women starting at 12 weeks of gestation.[1]

Anemia before conception or during pregnancy should be treated with 60 to 120 mg of ferrous iron per day, no more than about 60 mg per dose. A vitamin-mineral supplement containing 15 mg of zinc and 2 mg of copper was recommended to be taken at a different time of the day.[2] The hemoglobin should be checked for improvement after about 1 month, and the dose should be lowered to 30 mg/day if the anemia has resolved. The possibility of side effects was mentioned, including the likelihood that nausea, cramps, constipation, or diarrhea, should they develop, often persist for no longer than 3 to 5 days. Liquid and chewable preparations were offered as alternatives for women who have trouble swallowing pills or capsules. The relevant information provided about iron supplements is summarized in Table B-13.

Life Research Office: Guidelines for the Assessment and Management of Iron Deficiency in Women of Childbearing Age

This report (LSRO, 1991) focused primarily on the problem of iron deficiency in nonpregnant women. The recommendations for pregnant women were essentially the same as those of the Institute of Medicine (IOM, 1990a, 1992).

1. The prevalence of iron deficiency in the total population was considered to be sufficiently low to preclude recommending an increase in current levels of iron fortification in standardized food.

2. The prevalence of iron deficiency in nonpregnant women of childbearing age was too low to justify supplementing all women. Women with iron deficiency anemia should therefore be detected by laboratory screening, and intervention with iron supplements should be recommended for women with iron deficiency anemia.

3. Nonpregnant women should be screened for anemia (hemoglobin concentration, <12.0 g/dl, or hematocrit, <36 percent, with corrections for altitude and smoking [Table B-11]). For mild anemia (a hemoglobin concentration of between 10.0 and 12.0 g/dl), a therapeutic dose of iron, 60 mg twice a day, should be given for 6 weeks. Check for a change in hemoglobin concentration and continue for a total of 6 months, and then lower the dose to 30 mg/day and monitor iron status. For severe anemia (a hemoglobin concentration of <10.0 g/dl), investigate further for the cause of anemia (note that such low values are very rare). To make an etiologic diagnosis of anemia, serum ferritin concentra

---

[1] Note that recent developments argue for earlier initiation of iron or iron and folate: Studies indicate an association of anemia (Kim et al., 1992) or iron deficiency anemia (Scholl et al., 1992) early in pregnancy with low birth weight (IOM, 1992) and the CDC recommendations that all women of childbearing potential consume 0.4 mg of folate per day (CDC, 1992; IOM, 1992).

[2] The necessity for this recommendation might be reevaluated in light of evidence for decreased compliance when medication is recommended at intervals more frequent than once a day (IOM, 1992).

TABLE B-13 Information About Iron Supplements

Types of iron preparations
1. Well-absorbed iron compounds include ferrous sulfate, exsiccated ferrous sulfate, ferrous gluconate, and ferrous fumarate.
2. Slow-release iron compounds are available if there are side effects, but these are more expensive and are not as well absorbed.
3. Liquid and chewable preparations are available for those who have trouble swallowing tablets.
4. Iron compounds can be given alone, in combination with folate, or as part of a multivitamin-mineral combination, according to the clinical circumstances.
5. *Drug Facts and Comparisons* (Kastrup, 1992) is a useful, frequently updated reference for contents and costs of currently marketed iron products. It is available in many pharmacies and medical libraries.

Iron doses can be expressed in terms of elemental iron, as here, or in terms of the iron compound:
1. 30 mg of elemental iron is equivalent to:
   150 mg of ferrous sulfate
   about 95 mg of exsiccated ferrous sulfate
   90 mg of ferrous fumarate
   250 mg of ferrous gluconate
2. 60 mg of elemental iron is equivalent to:
   300 mg of ferrous sulfate
   about 190 mg of exsiccated ferrous sulfate
   180 mg of ferrous fumarate
   500 mg of ferrous gluconate

What to tell the patient to improve compliance and safety
1. Taking iron to prevent or treat iron deficiency anemia helps to reduce fatigue and increase your ability to adapt to delivery.
2. Let me give you the name of a liquid or chewable preparation if you have difficulty swallowing tablets.
3. Iron-containing supplements are best taken between meals or at bedtime with water or juice, not tea, coffee, or milk (once-a-day regimens favor compliance).
4. You may notice a darkening in the color of your stools, which normally results from taking iron tablets. Higher doses of iron sometimes cause stomach discomfort, constipation, or less often, diarrhea, but these problems often persist for no longer than the first 3 to 5 days after you start taking iron. If problems persist, we can lower the dose or recommend a different (slow-release) preparation that can be taken with meals.
5. Use safety caps (let me show you how), and keep supplements out of the reach of children because iron is a very common cause of poisoning (Litovitz et al., 1992).

SOURCE: IOM (1992).

tion determination is the preferred test. A value of less than 12 µg/liter by itself indicates iron deficiency. A value of less than 15 µg/liter in an anemic individual indicates iron deficiency anemia.

4. Therapeutic doses of iron for anemia should be given under medical supervision. The total daily dose can be between 60 and 180 mg/day but should not be more than about 60 mg per dose. Take iron alone with water or fruit juice, not with milk, tea, or coffee.

5. A maintenance dose of iron is 30 mg/day (range, 15 to 60 mg) when taken as prescribed (see discussion of RDAs below).

6. Advise on diet.

7. For follow-up, on a 6-week revisit, modify the dose according to the change in the hemoglobin concentration and compliance. Consider other causes of anemia if there has been no response.

8. Pregnant women should routinely take a maintenance dose of iron in the second and third trimesters even if they are not anemic. If anemic, they should receive a therapeutic dose of iron as described below. New CDC criteria for anemia during pregnancy should be used (Table B-11) (CDC, 1989).

Recommended Dietary Allowances, *10th Edition*

1. For nonpregnant women, 15 mg of iron per day was considered to provide a sufficient margin of safety for essentially all adult women in the United States except for those with the most extreme menstrual losses, given usual dietary patterns (NRC, 1989). This is a reduction from 18 mg/day in the 1980 RDAs.

2. For pregnant women, a daily increment of 15 mg/day (or a total of 30 mg/day) is recommended; this value is averaged over the entire pregnancy (NRC, 1989). Since the increased requirements of iron during pregnancy cannot be met by the iron content of the habitual diet of most Americans or the iron stores of at least some women, daily iron supplements are usually recommended.

Editorial Discussions

There is a widely held view in Britain (Hibbard, 1988) and elsewhere (Hemminki and Starfield, 1978) that no medication (including iron supplements) should be given to pregnant women in the absence of proven need. The view of Hemminki and coworkers (1989) was based on an earlier meta-analysis indicating no proven benefits of using vitamin or mineral supplements (Hemminki and Starfield, 1978). Hibbard (1988) proposed screening pregnant women and treating those in low-risk categories with iron only if they have a low serum ferritin concentration or anemia, but Horn (1988), in the same issue of the *British Medical Journal* as the article by Hibbard (1988), recommended routine iron supplementation as practical and cost-effective. Hibbard (1988) also recommended routine iron administration if concomitant folic acid treatment was used. Thus, the recent recommendation to use folate before conception and early in pregnancy would also include the use of iron if iron and folate combinations are prescribed, as is commonly the case.

International Recommendations Directed Primarily to Developing Countries

These recommendations are intended primarily for pregnant women in developing countries, where surveys have shown a prevalence of iron deficiency anemia often in excess of 50 percent (DeMaeyer et al., 1985). The recommendations have involved the routine use of relatively high doses of iron and folate. Poor distribution of tablets and poor compliance have been recognized as major problems. Various strategies for fortifying food with iron have been studied, but there has been little progress in implementing them on a broad scale.

FAO/WHO (1988) Requirements for absorbed iron were calculated for various age, sex, and pregnancy categories. Recommendations for dietary iron intakes are based on the estimated bioavailability of iron from the customary diet. The assumed percentage of iron absorbed primarily from cereal and legume diets, which have poor iron bioavailability, are 5 percent; that absorbed from diets with intermediate bioavailability, 10 percent; and that absorbed fromdiets with high bioavailability (meat and ascorbic acid-rich diets, as is usual in the United States), 15 percent.

World Health Organization The document *Preventing and Controlling Iron Deficiency Anemia Through Primary Health Care* (DeMaeyer, 1989) noted the need for supplementation in situations such as pregnancy, in which rapid improvement in iron status is important. It recognized the problem of compliance, especially when there may be side effects and no perception of ill health. It also stressed the need for communication and the importance of motivation skills for health workers. For pregnant women, the recommendation was to take tablets containing 60 mg of iron and 250 µg of folate twice a day. A diet rich in heme iron and ascorbic acid was advocated. The desirability of iron fortification of a staple food and the control of infection were discussed.

International Nutritional Anemia Consultative Group Tablets containing 60 mg of iron and 250 µg of folate twice a day without food were recommended for pregnant women. If there were side effects, the tablets were to be taken after meals or at a lower dose for 1 week before resuming a full dose. Diet modification and fortification were mentioned (INACG, 1989).

REFERENCES

AAP, CON (American Academy of Pediatrics, Committee on Nutrition). 1969. Iron balance and requirements in infancy. Pediatrics 43:134–142.
AAP, CON (American Academy of Pediatrics, Committee on Nutrition). 1976. Iron supplementation for infants. Pediatrics 58:765–768.
AAP, CON (American Academy of Pediatrics, Committee on Nutrition). 1985. Nutritional needs of low-birth-weight infants. Pediatrics 75:976–986.
AAP, CON (American Academy of Pediatrics, Committee on Nutrition). 1989. Iron-fortified infant formulas. Pediatrics 84:1114–1115.
AAP, CON (American Academy of Pediatrics, Committee on Nutrition). 1992. The use of whole cow's milk in infancy. Pediatrics 89:1105–1109.
AAP, CON (American Academy of Pediatrics, Committee on Nutrition). 1993. Pediatric Nutrition Handbook. Elk Grove, Ill: AAP.
ACOG (American College of Obstetricians and Gynecologists). 1989. Committee on Professional Standards. Standards for Obstetric-Gynecological Services, 7th ed. Washington, D.C.: ACOG.
AMA (American Medical Association). 1992. Guidelines for Adolescent Preventive Services. Report of the Department of Adolescent Health. Chicago: AMA.
Annest, J.L., J.L. Pirckle, D. Makue, J.W. Neese, D.D. Bayse, and M.G. Kovar. 1983. Chronological trend in blood lead levels between 1976 and 1980. N. Engl. J. Med. 308:1373–1377.
Babior, B.M., W.A. Peters, P.M. Briden, and C.L. Cetrulo. 1985. Pregnant women's absorption of iron from prenatal supplements. J. Reprod. Med. 30:355–357.
Beutler, E. 1988. The common anemias. J. Am. Med. Assoc. 259:2433–2437.
Bonnar, J., A. Goldberg, and J.A. Smith. 1969. Do pregnant women take their iron? Lancet 1:457–458.
Bothwell, T.H., and R.W. Charlton. 1981. Iron Deficiency in Women. Washington, D.C.: International Nutrition Anemia Consultative Group.
Bothwell, T.H., and P. Macphail. 1992. Prevention of iron deficiency by food fortification. Pp. 183–192 in Nutritional Anemias, S.J. Fomon and S. Zlotkin, eds. Nestlé Nutrition Workshop Series, Vol. 30. New York: Raven Press.
Bothwell, T.H., R.W. Charlton, J.D. Cook, and C.A. Finch. 1979. Iron Metabolism in Man. Blackwell: Oxford.
Bothwell, T.H., R.D. Baynes, B.J. MacFarlane, and A.P. MacPhail. 1989. Nutritional iron requirements and food iron absorption. J. Int. Med. 226:357–365.
Calvo, E.B., A.C. Galindo, and N.B. Aspres. 1992. Iron status in exclusively breast-fed infants. Pediatrics 90:375–379.
Canadian Paediatric Society, Nutrition Committee. 1991. Meeting the iron needs of infants and young children: An update. Can. Med. Assoc. J. 144:1451–1453.
Carriaga, M.T., B.S. Skikne, B. Finley, B. Cutler, and J.D. Cook. 1991. Serum transferrin receptor for the detection of iron deficiency in pregnancy. Am. J. Clin. Nutr. 54:1077–1081.
CDC (Centers for Disease Control). 1989. CDC criteria for anemia in children and childbearing-aged women. Morbid. Mortal. Weekly Rep. 38:400–404.
CDC (Centers for Disease Control). 1992. Recommendations for the use of folic acid to reduce the number of cases of spina bifida and other neural tube defects. Morbid. Mortal. Weekly Rep. 41(No. RR-14):1–7.

Chanarin, I., and D. Rothman. 1971. Further observations on the relation between iron and folate status in pregnancy. Br. Med. J. 2:81–84.

Charlton, R.W., and T.H. Bothwell. 1983. Iron absorption. Annu. Rev. Med. 34:55–68.

Clapp, J.F., B.L. Seaward, R.H. Sleamaker, and J. Hiser. 1988. Maternal physiologic adaptations to early pregnancy. Am. J. Obstet Gynecol. 159:1456–1460.

Clark, M., R. Royal, and R. Seeler. 1988. Interaction of iron deficiency and lead and the hematologic findings in children with severe lead poisoning. Pediatrics 81:247–254.

Cook, J.D. 1990. Adaptation in iron metabolism. Am. J. Clin. Nutr. 51:301–308.

Cook, J.D., and T.H. Bothwell. 1984. Availability of iron from infant food. Pp. 119–143 in Nutrition in Infancy and Childhood, A. Stekel, ed. New York: Raven Press.

Cook, J.D., C.A. Finch, and N.J. Smith. 1976. Evaluation of the iron status of a population. Blood 48:449–455.

Cook, J.D., S.S. Watson, K.M. Simpson, D.A. Lipschitz, and B.S. Skigne. 1984. The effect of high ascorbic acid supplementation on body iron stores. Blood 64:721–726.

Cook, J.D., S.A. Dassenko, and S.R. Lynch. 1991. Assessment of the role of nonheme-iron availability in iron balance. Am. J. Clin. Nutr. 54:717–722.

Cook, J.D., B.S. Skikme, and R.D. Baynes. 1993. Serum transferrin receptor. Annu. Rev. Med. 44:63–74.

Cramer, J.A., R.H. Mattson, M.L. Prevey, R.D. Scheyer, and V.L. Ouellette. 1989. How often is medication taken as prescribed? A novel assessment technique. J. Am. Med. Assoc. 261:3273–3277.

Cramer, J.A., R.D. Scheyer, and R.H. Mattson. 1990. Compliance declines between clinic visits. Arch. Intern. Med. 150:1509–1510.

Crosby, W.H. 1986. Yin, yang, and iron. Nutrition Today July/Aug:14–16.

Cross, C.E., B. Halliwell, E.T. Borish, W.A. Pryor, R.L. Saul, J.M. McDord, and D. Harman. 1987. Oxygen radicals and human disease. Ann. Intern. Med. 107:526–545.

Czeizel, A.E., and I. Dudas. 1992. Prevention of the first occurrence of neural-tube defects by periconceptual vitamin supplementation. N. Engl. J. Med. 327:1832–1835.

Dallman, P.R. 1986. Biochemical basis for manifestations of iron deficiency. Annu. Rev. Nutr. 6:13–40.

Dallman, P.R. 1987. Iron deficiency and the immune response. Am. J. Clin. Nutr. 46:329–334.

Dallman, P.R. 1988. Nutritional anemia of infancy: Iron, folic acid, and vitamin B_{12}. Pp. 216–235 in Nutrition During Infancy, R.C. Tsang and B.L. Nichols, eds. Philadelphia: Hanley and Belfus.

Dallman, P.R. 1992. Changing iron needs from birth through adolescence. Pp. 29–36 in Nutritional Anemias, S.J. Fomon and S. Zlotkin, eds. New York: Raven Press.

Dallman, P.R., and J.D. Reeves. 1984. Laboratory diagnosis of iron deficiency. Pp. 11–44 in Nutrition in Infancy and Childhood, A. Stekel, ed. New York: Raven Press.

Dallman, P.R., and M.A. Siimes. 1979. Percentile curves for hemoglobin and red cell volume in infancy and childhood. J. Pediatr. 94:26–31.

Dallman, P.R., G.D. Barr, C.M. Allen, and H.R. Shinefield. 1978. Hemoglobin concentration in white, black, and Oriental children: is there a need for separate criteria in screening for anemia? Am. J. Clin. Nutr. 31:377–380.

Dawson, E.B., and W.J. McGanity. 1987. Protection of maternal iron stores in pregnancy. J. Reprod. Med. 32:478–487.

DeMaeyer, E.M. 1989. Preventing and Controlling Iron Deficiency Anaemia Through Primary Health Care. Geneva: World Health Organization.

DeMaeyer, E.M., M. Adiels-Tegman, and E. Rayston. 1985. The prevalence of anemia in the world. World Health Statist. Q. 38:302–316.

DHHS/USDA (U.S. Department of Health and Human Services and U.S. Department of Agriculture). 1991. Nutrition and Your Health: Dietary Guidelines for Americans, 3rd ed. Washington, D.C.: U.S. Government Printing Office.

Duncan, B., R.B. Schifman, J.J. Corrigan, and C. Schaefer. 1985. Iron and the exclusively breast-fed infant from birth to six months. J. Pediatr. Gastroenterol. Nutr. 4:421–425.

Ekenved, G., B. Arvidsson, and L. Sölvell. 1976. Influence of food on the absorption from different types of iron tablets. Scand. J. Haematol. 28(Suppl.):79–88.

Expert Scientific Working Group. 1985. Summary of a report on assessment of the iron nutritional status of the United States population. Am. J. Clin. Nutr. 42:1318–1330.

FAO/WHO (Food and Agriculture Organization of the United Nations/World Health Organization). 1988. 1988 Report of a Joint FAO/WHO Expert Consultation. Pp. 33–50 in Requirements of Vitamin A, Iron, Folate and Vitamin B_{12}. Rome: Food and Agriculture Organization of the United Nations.

Ferguson, B.J., B.S. Skigne, K.M. Simpson, R.D. Baynes, and J.D. Cook. 1992. Serum transferrin receptor distinguishes the anemia of chronic from iron deficiency anemia. J. Lab. Clin. Med. 119:385–390.

Fomon, S.J. 1987. Reflections on infant feeding in the 1970s and 1980s. Am. J. Clin. Nutr. 46:171–182.

Fomon, S.J., E.E. Ziegler, R.R. Rogers, S.E. Nelson, B.B. Edwards, D.G. Guy, J.C. Erve, and M. Janghorbani. 1989. Iron absorption from infant foods. Pediatr. Res. 26:250–254.

Galan, P., F. Cherouvrier, P. Preziosi, and S. Hercberg. 1991. Effects of the increased consumption of dairy products upon iron absorption. Eur. J. Clin. Nutr. 45:553–559.

Garn, S.M., S.A. Ridella, A.S. Tetzold, and F. Falkner. 1981. Maternal hematological levels and pregnancy outcomes. Semin. Perinatol. 5:155–162.

Groner, J.A., N.A. Holtzman, E. Charney, and D.E. Mellits. 1986. A randomized trial of oral iron on tests of short-term memory and attention span in young pregnant women. J. Adolescent Health Care 7:44–48.

Hahn, P.F., E.L. Carothers, W.J. Darby, M. Martin, C.W. Sheppard, R.O. Cannon, A.S. Beam, P.M. Denson, J.C. Peterson, and G.S. McClellan. 1951. Iron metabolism in human pregnancy as studied with the radioactive isotope, Fe^{59}. Am. J. Obstet. Gynecol. 61:477–486.

Hallberg, L. 1981. Bioavailability of dietary iron in man. Annu. Rev. Nutr. 1:123–147.

Hallberg, L. 1992. Iron requirements. Comments on methods and some crucial concepts in iron nutrition. Biol. Trace Elements Res. 35:25–45.

Hallberg, L. 1988. Iron balance in pregnancy. Pp 115–126 in Vitamins and Minerals in Pregnancy and Lactation, H. Berger, ed. Nestlé Nutrition Workshop Series, Vol. 16. New York: Raven Press.

Hallberg, L., and L. Rossander. 1982. Absorption of iron from Western-type lunch and dinner meals. Am. J. Clin. Nutr. 35:502–509.

Hallberg, L., A.M. Högdahl, L. Nilsson, and G. Rybo. 1966. Menstrual blood loss—a population study. Variation at different ages and attempts to define normality. Acta Obstet. Gynecol. Scand. 45:320–351.

Hallberg, L., L. Ryttinger, and L. Sölvell. 1967. Side effects of oral iron therapy: A double-blind study of different iron compounds in tablet form. Acta Med. Scand. Suppl. 459:3–10.

Hallberg, L., M. Brune, M. Erlandsson, A.-S. Sandberg, and L. Rossander-Hultén. 1991. Calcium: Effect of different amounts on nonheme- and heme-iron absorption in humans. Am. J. Clin. Nutr. 53:112–119.

Hallberg, L., L. Rossander-Hulten, M. Brune, and A. Gleerup. 1992. Bioavailability of iron in human milk and cow's milk in relation to their calcium contents. Pediatr. Res. 31:524–527.

Hallberg, L., L. Hulten, G. Lindstedt, P.-A. Lunberg, M. Anders, J. Purens, B. Svanberg, and B. Swolin. In press. High prevalence of iron deficiency in Swedish adolescents. Pediatr. Res.

Hambidge, K.M., N.F. Krebs, L. Sibley, and J. English. 1987. Acute effects of iron therapy on zinc status during pregnancy. Obstet. Gynecol. 70:593–596.

Haynes, R.B. 1979. Strategies for improving compliance: A methodologic analysis and review. Pp 69–82 in Compliance in Health Care, R.B. Haynes, D.W. Taylor, and D.L. Sackett, eds. Baltimore: Johns Hopkins University Press.

Haynes, R.B., D.W. Taylor, and D.L. Sackett, eds. 1979. Compliance in Health Care. Baltimore: Johns Hopkins University Press.

Hemminki, E., and B. Starfield. 1978. Routine administration of iron and vitamins during pregnancy: Review of controlled clinical trials. Br. J. Obstet. Gynaecol. 85:404–410.

Hibbard, B.M. 1988. Controversies in therapeutics. Iron and folate supplements during pregnancy: Supplementation is valuable only in selected patients. Br. Med. J. 297:1324–1326.

Horn, E. 1988. Controversies in therapeutics. Iron and folate supplements during pregnancy: Supplementing everyone treats those at risk and is cost effective. Br. Med. J. 297:1325–1327.

Hurrell, R.F. 1992. Prospects for improving the iron fortification of foods. Pp. 193–201 in Nutritional Anemias, S.J. Fomon and S. Zlotkin, eds. Nestlé Nutrition Workshop Series, Vol. 30. New York: Raven Press.

Idjradinata, P., and E. Pollitt. 1993. Reversal of developmental delays in iron-deficient anaemic infants treated with iron. Lancet 341:1–4.

INACG (International Nutritional Anemia Consultative Group). 1989. Guidelines for the Control of Maternal Nutritional Anemia. International Life Sciences Institute-Nutrition Foundation. Washington, D.C.: INACG.

IOM (Institute of Medicine). 1990a. Nutrition During Pregnancy. Report of the Committee on Nutritional Status During Pregnancy and Lactation, Food and Nutrition Board. Washington, D.C.: National Academy Press.

IOM (Institute of Medicine). 1990b. Iron nutrition during pregnancy. Pp. 272–298 in Nutrition During Pregnancy. Report of the Committee on Nutritional Status During Pregnancy and Lactation, Food and Nutrition Board. Washington, D.C.: National Academy Press.

IOM (Institute of Medicine). 1992. Nutrition During Pregnancy and Lactation: An Implementation Guide. Report of the Subcommittee for a Clinical Application Guide, Committee on Nutritional Status During Pregnancy and Lactation, Food and Nutrition Board. Washington, D.C.: National Academy Press.

Johnson-Spear, M.A., and R. Yip. In press. Hemoglobin difference between black and white women with comparable iron status: Justification for race-specific criteria? Am. J. Clin. Nutr.

Kastrup, E.K., ed. 1992. Drug Facts and Comparisons. St. Louis: Facts and Comparisons.

Kim, I., D.W. Hungerford, R. Yip, S.A. Kuester, C. Zyrkowski, and F.L. Trowbridge. 1992. Pregnancy nutrition surveillance system—United States, 1979–1990. CDC Surveillance Summaries. Morbid. Mortal. Weekly Rep. 41(No. SS-7):26–42.

Laplan, J.P., J.L. Annest, P.M. Layde, and G.L. Rubin. 1986. Nutrient intake and supplementation in the United States (NHANES II). Am. J. Public Health 76:287–289.

Litovitz, T.L., K.C. Holm, K.M. Bailey, and B.F. Schmitz. 1992. 1991 Annual report of the American Association of Poison Control Centers National Data Collection System. Am. J. Emerg. Med. 10:452–505.

Looker, A.C., C. L. Johnson, M.A. McDowell, and E.A. Yetley. 1989. Iron status: Prevalence of impairment in three Hispanic groups in the United States. Am. J. Clin. Nutr. 49:553–558.

Lozoff, B., E. Jimenez, and A.B. Wolf. 1991. Long-term developmental outcome of infants with iron deficiency. N. Engl. J. Med. 325:687–694.

LSRO (Life Sciences Research Office). 1984. Assessment of the Iron Nutritional Status of the U.S. Population Based on Data Collected in the Second National Health and Nutrition Examination Survey, 1976–1980. Bethesda, Md.: Federation of American Societies for Experimental Biology.

LSRO (Life Sciences Research Office). 1989. Nutrition Monitoring in the United States—An Update Report on Nutrition Monitoring. DHHS Publication No. (PHS) 89-1255. Public Health Service. Washington, D.C.: U.S. Government Printing Office.

LSRO (Life Sciences Research Office). 1991. Guidelines for the Assessment and Management of Iron Deficiency in Women of Childbearing Age, S.A. Anderson, ed. Bethesda, Md.: Federation of American Societies for Experimental Biology.

Lundström, U., M.A. Siimes, and P.R. Dallman. 1977. At what age does iron supplementation become necessary in low-birth-weight infants? J. Pediatr. 91:878–883.

Monsen, E.R., L. Hallberg, M. Layrisse, D.M. Hegsted, J.D. Cook, W. Mertz, and C.A. Finch. 1978. Estimation of available dietary iron. Am. J. Clin. Nutr. 31:134–141.

Murphy, J.F., J. O'Riordan, R.G. Newcombe, and E.C. Coles. 1986. Relation of haemoglobin levels in first and second trimesters to outcome of pregnancy. Lancet 1:992–994.

NRC (National Research Council). 1989. Recommended Dietary Allowances, 10th ed. Report of the Subcommittee on the Tenth Edition of the RDAs, Food and Nutrition Board, Commission of Life Sciences. Washington, D.C.: National Academy Press.

Penrod, J.C., K. Anderson, and P.B. Acosta. 1990. Impact on iron status of introducing cow's milk in the second six months of life. J. Pediatr. Gastroenterol. Nutr. 10:462–467.

Perry, G.S., T. Byers, R. Yip, and S. Margen. 1992. Iron nutrition does not account for hemoglobin differences between blacks and whites. J. Nutr. 122:1417–1424.

Pizarro, F., R. Yip, P.R. Dallman, M. Olivares, E. Hertrampf, and R. Walter. 1991. Iron status with different infant feeding regimens: Relevance to screening and prevention of iron deficiency. J. Pediatr. 118:687–692.

Pollitt, E., P. Hathirat, N.J. Kotchabhakdi, L. Missell, and A. Valyasevi. 1989. Iron deficiency and educational achievement in Thailand. Am. J. Clin. Nutr. 50:687–697.

Porter, A.M.W. 1969. Drug defaulting in a general practice. Br. Med. J. 1:218–222.

Puolakka, J., O. Jänne, A. Pakarinen, and R. Vihko. 1980. Serum ferritin as a measure of stores during and after normal pregnancy with and without iron supplements. Acta Obstet. Gynecol Scand. Suppl. 95:43–51.

Reeves, J.D., R. Yip, V. Kiley, and P.R. Dallman. 1984. Iron deficiency in infants, the influence of antecedent infection. J. Pediatr. 105:874–879.

Romslo, I., K. Haram, N. Sagen, and K. Augensen. 1983. Iron requirements in normal pregnancy as assessed by serum ferritin, serum transferrin saturation, and erythrocyte protoporphyrin determinations. Br. J. Obstet. Gynaecol. 90:101–107.

Rossander, L., L. Hallberg, and E. Björn-Rasmussen. 1979. Absorption of iron from breakfast meals. Am. J. Clin. Nutr. 32:2484–2489.

Salonen, J.T., K. Nyyssönen, H. Korpela, J. Tuomilehto, R. Seppänen, and R. Salonen. 1992. High stored iron levels are associated with excess risk of myocardial infarction in Eastern Finnish men. Circulation 86:803–811.

Schifman, R.B., J.E. Thomasson, and J.M. Evers. 1987. Red blood cell zinc protoporphyrin testing for iron-deficiency anemia in pregnancy. Am. J. Obstet. Gynecol. 157:304–307.

Scholl, T.O., M.L. Hediger, R.L. Fischer, and J.W. Shearer. 1992. Anemia vs. iron deficiency: Increased risk of preterm delivery in a prospective study. Am. J. Clin. Nutr. 55:985–988.

Seligman, P.A., J.H. Caskey, J.L. Frazier, R.M. Zucker, E.R. Podell, and R.H. Allen. 1983. Measurements of iron absorption from prenatal multivitamin-mineral supplements. Obstet. Gynecol. 61:356–362.

Sheldon, W.L., M.O. Aspillaga, P.A. Smith, and T. Lind. 1985. The effects of oral iron supplementation on zinc and magnesium levels during pregnancy. Br. J. Obstet. Gynaecol. 92:892–898.

Siegenberg, D., R.D. Baynes, T.H. Bothwell, B.J. MacFarlane, R.D. Lamparelli, N.G. Car, P. McPhail, U. Schmidt, A. Tal, and F. Mayet. 1991. Ascorbic acid prevents the dose dependent inhibitory effects of polyphenols and phytates on non-heme iron absorption. Am. J. Clin. Nutr. 53:537–541.

Siimes, M.A., L. Salmenperä, and J. Perheentupa. 1984. Exclusively breast-feeding for nine months: Risk of iron deficiency. J. Pediatr. 104:196–199.

Sjöstedt, J.E., P. Manner, S. Nummi, and G. Ekenved. 1977. Oral iron prophylaxis during pregnancy: A comparative study on different dosage regimens. Acta Obstet. Gynecol. Scand. Suppl. 60:3–9.

Sölvell, L. 1970. Oral iron therapy-side effects. Pp. 573–583 in Iron Deficiency: Pathogenesis, Clinical Aspects, Therapy, L. Hallberg, H.G. Harwerth, and A. Vannotti, eds. London: Academic Press.

Subar, A.F., and G. Block. 1990. Use of vitamin and mineral supplements: Demographics and amounts of nutrients consumed. Am J. Epidemiol. 132:1091–1101.

Svanberg, B., B. Arvidsson, A. Norrby, G. Rybo, and L. Sölvell. 1976. Absorption of supplemental iron during pregnancy—A longitudinal study with repeated bone-marrow studies and absorption measurements. Acta Obstet. Gynecol. Scand. Suppl. 48:87–108.

Swiss, L.D., and G.H. Beaton. 1974. A prediction of the effects of iron fortification. Am. J. Clin. Nutr. 27:373–379.

Taylor, D.J., C. Mallen, N. McDougall, and T. Lind. 1982. Effect of iron supplementation on serum ferritin levels during and after pregnancy. Br. J. Obstet. Gynecol. 89:1011–1017.

Tunnessen, W.W., and F.A. Oski. 1987. Consequences of starting whole cow milk at 6 months of age. J. Pediatr. 111:813–816.

Uchida, T., M. Yoshida, K. Sakai, K. Kokubun, T. Igarashi, T. Tanaka, and S. Kariyone. 1988. Prevalence of iron deficiency in Japanese women. Acta Haematol. Jpn. 51:24–27.

Ulmer, H.U., and E. Goepel. 1988. Anemia, ferritin and preterm labor. J. Perinat. Med. 16:459–465.

Wallenburg, H.C.S., and H.G. van Eijk. 1984. Effect of oral iron supplementation during pregnancy on maternal and fetal iron status. J. Perinat. Med. 12:7–11.

Walter, T., I. De Andraca, P. Chadud, and C.G. Perales. 1989. Iron deficiency anemia: Adverse effects on infant psychomotor development. Pediatrics 84:7–17.

Walter, T., P.R. Dallman, F. Pizarro, L. Veloso, G. Peña, S. Bartholmey, E. Hertrampf, M. Olivares, A. Letelier, and M. Arredondo. 1993. Effectiveness of iron-fortified infant cereal in prevention of iron deficiency anemia. Pediatrics 91:976–982.

Weinberg, E.D. 1984. Iron withholding. Physiol. Rev. 64:65–102.

Weinberg, E.D. 1992. Roles of iron in neoplasia. Biol. Trace Element Res. 34:123–140.

Widholm, O., E. Vartiainen, and T. Tenhunen. 1967. On iron requirements in menstruating teen-age girls. Acta Obstet. Gynecol. Scand. 46(Suppl. 1):31–46.

Yip, R. 1989. The changing characteristics of childhood iron nutritional status in the United States. Pp. 37–56 in Dietary Iron: Birth to Two Years, L.J. Filer, Jr., ed. New York: Raven Press.

Yip, R., S. Schwartz, and A.S. Deinard. 1984. Hematocrit values in white, black, and American Indian children with comparable iron status: Evidence to support uniform diagnostic criteria for anemia among all races. Am. J. Dis. Child. 138:824–827.

Yip, R., K.M. Walsh, M.G. Goldfarb, and N.J. Binkin. 1987a. Declining prevalence of anemia in childhood in a middle-class setting: A pediatric success story? Pediatrics 80:330–334.

Yip, R., N.J. Binkin, L. Fleshood, and F.L. Trowbridge. 1987b. Declining prevalence of anemia among low-income children in the United States. J. Am. Med. Assoc. 258:1619–1623.

Ziegler, E.E., S.J. Fomon, S.E. Nelson, C.J. Rebouche, B.B. Edwards, R.R. Rogers, and L.J. Lehman. 1990. Cow milk feeding in infancy: Further observations on blood loss from the gastrointestinal tract. J. Pediatr. 116:11–18.

C

Iron-Dependent Pathologies

John L. Beard [1]

A recent article by Salonen and colleagues in *Circulation* has sparked the interest of a number of individuals both within and outside of the scientific community (Salonen et al., 1992). The research question posed by the authors and suggested by a growing number of observations was relatively straightforward: Is excess body iron, as indicated by the plasma ferritin concentration, a significant positive risk factor for myocardial infarction? The biologic feasibility of this question has its roots in the reasonably well established in vitro relationships between free-radical production and iron content in physiologic solutions (Halliwell and Gutteridge, 1990; Reif, 1992). The Haber-Weiss reaction (equation 1)

$$O_2 \bullet + H_2O_2 \rightarrow O_2 OH^- + OH \bullet \tag{1}$$

can be modified in the presence of Fe^{+3} to a much faster set of reactions (equations 2 and 3) called the *Fenton reaction*:

$$O_2 + Fe^{+3} \rightarrow O_2 + Fe^{+2} \tag{2}$$

$$Fe^{+2} + H_2O_2 \rightarrow Fe^{+3} + OH^- + OH \bullet \tag{3}$$

The hypotheses concerning the effect of the chronic toxicity of iron with regard to its relationship with cancer, atherosclerosis, and neurodegenerative disorders have a common theme in the iron-catalyzed production of highly reactive oxygen species. A recent census lists 60 human diseases in which oxidant stress is thought to play a role (Halliwell, 1987).

Although it is true that iron can catalyze a number of biologically undesirable reactions in vitro, iron is nearly always chelated to low-molecular-weight compounds or is associated with macromolecules such as proteins, lipids, carbohydrates, and nucleic acids in vivo and under nonpathologic conditions. Free

---

[1] The author acknowledges the assistance of Harry Dawson in the literature review for sections of this paper as well as the contribution of James Connor for material on the brain pathology sections.

iron can be liberated by redox reagents from iron-protein complexes but is frequently oxidized to the ferric state by ceruloplasmin (Gutteridge, 1986; Gutteridge et al., 1980). Recent evidence obtained by electromagnetic proton resonance suggests that the Fenton reaction occurs only when plasma is exposed to atmospheric oxygen and that even iron-overloaded plasma does not produce the superoxide-driven Fenton reaction (Minetti et al., 1992). Some authors have suggested that an endogenous pool of low-molecular-weight proteins such as di- and trinucleotides, citrate, acetate, and urate complexed to ferrous iron are sources of hydroxyl radicals (Floyd, 1983).

The highly reactive product oxidant molecules are the sources of extensive oxidative stress to cellular systems and are the basis of extensive studies by Halliwell and Gutteridge (1990). The sources of this "free iron" in vivo are unknown at this time, and the in vivo locations are undetermined. Oxidized iron is transported in a tightly bound fashion to transferrin in the plasma pool and is not readily removed by most endogenous or exogenous chelators of iron unless the pH drops significantly below 6.0. Thus, the amount of free iron in plasma in normal physiologic states is extremely low and is an unlikely source of iron for the Fenton reaction. A second possible source of iron in the plasma pool or in cells is ferritin (Reif, 1992). Apoferritin is composed of 24 protein subunits containing either heavy or light chains. The heavy-chain subunit has considerable ferroxidase activity, whereas the amounts of both chains regulate the rate of entry and exodus of ferric iron from its ferric oxide core (Cozzi et al., 1990; Craelius et al., 1974). Ferritin is usually less than 20 percent saturated with iron while in the plasma compartment. The iron in fully loaded ferritin is more labile than that in normally loaded ferritin (Gutteridge et al., 1983). In vitro studies have frequently driven the mobilization of this ferritin-bound iron by adding supraphysiologic amounts of oxidants, chelators, and iron-loaded ferritin. A number of compounds with a reducing potential in excess of -230 mV can remove ferritin-bound iron at physiologic pH. Unfortunately, most in vitro studies have used chelators and oxidizing agents that have iron-binding affinities in excess of those likely to exist for in vivo chelators (Reif, 1992). The presence of appropriate antioxidants can prevent this iron removal. Thomas and colleagues (1985) and others (Gutteridge et al., 1983) have shown increased lipid peroxidation when iron is released from ferritin. The extent of damage can be limited by the addition of iron chelators such as desferoxamine, although its binding affinity for iron (10^{31}) is much higher than those of other likely in vivo chelators.

The redox potential for superoxide (0.33 mV) suggests that superoxide is capable of reducing the ferric iron core of ferritin (Crighton et al., 1980). This superoxide is generated in vivo by xanthine oxidase during respiratory bursts by neutrophils and during reperfusion injury of ischemic tissues (Bolann and Ulvik, 1990). Although superoxide is able to mobilize few ferrous iron atoms in normally saturated ferritin, the number increases 3.5-fold by the addition of the chelator EDTA. Other studies show that the iron liberated from ferritin by superoxide can be scavenged by both transferrin and lactoferrin or reoxidized by ceruloplasmin in vitro (Monteiro and Winterbourn, 1988; Samokyszyn et al., 1989, 1991). Transferrin and lactoferrin are unlikely donators given their high binding affinity for iron (10^{24}) at physiologic pH. In contrast, transferrin and lactoferrin inhibit iron-catalyzed lipid peroxidation in vitro (Gutteridge et al., 1981). Heme iron can be removed by oxidants such as H_2O_2 in vitro (Puppo and Halliwell, 1988). This can cause cytotoxicity in cells exposed to both heme and oxidant stress. Hemopexin and haptoglobin complexes with hemoglobin both act to prevent lipid peroxidation (Gutteridge, 1987).

The direct evidence for free iron availability comes from the bleomycin-reactive iron assay or inhibition of reactions by the iron chelator desferoxamine. Bleomycin-detectable iron is absent from the plasma, serum, and synovial fluid of healthy adult individuals. It can be found in the plasma of premature and full-term neonates, with higher levels occurring in the premature neonate group (Evans et al., 1992). These levels correspond to the ability of surfactant from neonates to induce lipid peroxidation (Moison et al., 1993). Bleomycin-detectable iron is also found in the plasma and synovial fluid of patients with idiopathic hemochromatosis, bone marrow transplant recipients, and patients with acute nonlymphocytic leukemia (Foerder et al., 1992; Gordeuk and Brittenham, 1992; Gutteridge, 1992; Pillay and Makgoba, 1992). This free iron has also been found in the gruel of atherosclerotic lesions (Smith et al., 1992).

HEART DISEASE

The oxidation of low-density lipoproteins (LDLs) has been experimentally related to the presence of iron (Kuzuya et al., 1990; Steinberg et al., 1989). An increased proportion of LDLs was oxidized after exposure to high levels of iron, and there was a more rapid uptake of LDLs into cells. It is the rapid and relatively uncontrolled uptake of these oxidized LDLs that are key elements in the current hypothesis of the pathogenesis of coronary heart disease (CHD) (Steinberg et al., 1989).

The study by Salonen and colleagues (1992) that has caused such recent public concern was a prospective examination of novel risk factors for acute myocardial infarction and atherogenesis (AMI). The subject population was a group of 3,235 eastern Finnish men who were enrolled in the study at ages 42, 48, 54, and 60 years and who were followed for 5 years. The authors established by a proportional hazards model that an elevated plasma ferritin concentration was one of the significant factors for AMI after a statistical adjustment for age and year of enrollment. The relative risk was 2.2 for men with a serum ferritin concentration of 200 µg/liter or greater. Further separation of the elevated ferritin group into groups with serum ferritin concentrations of 200–400 and greater than 400 µg/liter did not change the risk ratio, indicating an effect well within a range of ferritin concentrations at the high end of normal. The men who had heart attacks had a higher mean ferritin concentration (231 ± 215 µg/liter) than those who did not (165 ± 146 µg/liter). It is important to note that equal numbers of men with serum ferritin concentrations of less than 200 µg/liter and greater than 200 µg/liter had heart attacks. The authors noted that a significant difference persists between these two groups after a covariance adjustment is made on the basis of other risk factors such as lipoprotein concentrations and smoking history. The distribution of serum ferritin concentrations showed that about 10 percent of the men in their fourth and fifth decades of life had a serum ferritin concentration of greater than 280 µg/liter. This percentage is comparable to that reported by Salonen and colleagues (1992) for the non-AMI portion of the sample and is a considerably lower percentage than that in the AMI sample (18 percent). Thus, although the non-AMI sample had a distribution similar to that in the U.S. population, the AMI group appeared to be shifted to the right of the mean and to have a small group of subjects with extremely high serum ferritin concentrations. A recent estimate of the prevalence of the hemochromatosis gene defect in Europe and the United States is that 4.5 people per 1,000 population are homozygous, and about 12.5 percent of the population is estimated to be heterozygous. Although the gene prevalence in the sample population is not known, it is possible that this iron-loading gene defect plays a significant role in the established statistical relationship. Previous reports demonstrate a low prevalence of less than 1/1,000 population in other parts of Finland, but also recognize that pockets of increased prevalence may exist in the Finnish population (Karlsson et al., 1988). Near the upper end of the ferritin distribution, the transferrin saturation can approach 100 percent (Bothwell and Charlton, 1982). It is at this point that free iron may be present in plasma and act in the aforementioned manner as a participant in the Haber-Weiss reaction (Aruoma et al., 1988). Congestive heart failure is characteristic of hereditary hemochromatosis and is prevented by chelation or phlebotomy. Recent evidence in the reperfusion-ischemia literature demonstrates a strong role for chelatable iron in the initiation of cellular oxidative damage (Van der Kraaij et al., 1988; Williams et al., 1991).

The positive effects of ferritin on oxidation-mediated damage, however, should be considered. Apoferritin added to cultured endothelial cells protects them from oxidant-mediated cytolysis because of its strong ferroxidase affinity (Balla et al., 1991). The antioxidant status of the microenvironment in vivo may ultimately determine whether iron-catalyzed oxidative damage to LDLs is a significant component of atherogenesis. In a prospective study of U.S. physicians, an increased risk (relative risk of 1.1) was reported for those with a high level of serum ferritin, although dietary iron had no relationship to risk of CHD (Rimm et al., 1993). This does not support the hypothesis that dietary iron increases coronary risk in men, nor is it consistent with a 5 percent increase in the risk of CHD with a 1-mg increase in iron intake per day, as suggested by Salonen and colleagues (1992).

CANCER

The experimental evidence relating iron status to carcinogenesis is usually derived from studies that use very large quantities of iron. For example, mammary carcinogenesis induced by 1-methyl-nitrosourea is increased in rats fed 1,200 mg/ml of iron compared with that in rats fed 20 or 2 mg/ml (Thompson et al., 1991). In a model of induced mammary carcinogenesis, mice fed 5 mg/kg of iron developed tumors at a faster rate than mice fed iron at 180 mg/kg. There was no increase in overall tumor incidence. Iron potentiates 1,2-dimethyhydrazine-induced colon cancer (20 mg/kg) at a level of 3.5 percent ferrous fumarate (11,504 mg/kg of elemental iron) in the diet (Siegers et al., 1988, 1992). Experimental iron deficiency is associated with delayed onset time of experimental liver tumors (Vitale et al., 1977), whereas choline-deficient rats fed a low-iron diet developed fewer preneoplastic liver lesions than rats fed 330 mg/kg of iron (Yoshigi et al., 1992).

In a screening designed to assess the carcinogenicity of pharmaceutical preparations, an increased risk of lung cancer was noted among male users of nonprenatal iron formulations (Friedman and Ury, 1980, 1983). A 24-hour recall survey of the Transkei region of South Africa found a significant increase in intake of dietary iron among those at increased risk of esophageal cancer (Groenwald et al., 1981). In a retrospective case-control study of 186 subjects, iron consumption varied inversely with the size of colonic polyps but showed no correlation with the size of the initial dysplasia (Hoff et al., 1986). A prospective study of colorectal cancer in Majorca concluded that the daily iron intake was greater in females who developed colon cancer than in population controls (Benito, 1991). Data from the first National Health and Nutrition Examination Survey indicate that the total iron-binding capacity is lower and the transferrin saturation is higher among men who developed cancer (Stevens et al., 1988). An association in women was evident only at extremely high transferrin saturations. Similar and opposite relationships affected by gender are evident in other studies (Selby and Friedman, 1988; Stevens et al., 1986). It is not clear whether these data clarify any role in the pathogenesis of iron-related carcinogenesis.

BRAIN IRON AND DISEASE

A number of neurologic disorders, including Parkinson's disease (Olanow et al., 1992), multiple sclerosis (Drayer et al., 1987), Alzheimer's disease (Connor, 1992), and Hallervorden-Spatz disease (Swaiman, 1991), are associated with disruptions in iron homeostasis in the brain. It is clear that normal neurologic function is dependent on normal iron homeostasis. The brain has the highest rate of oxidative metabolism of any organ in the body, which probably accounts for the finding that levels of iron are higher in the brain that in any organ except the liver (Hallgren and Sourander, 1958).

Parkinson's Disease

Research attention has focused on the involvement of iron in neurologic disease, particularly as it relates to oxidative damage. Data describing the postmortem brain iron contents of individuals who had Parkinson's disease (Sofic et al., 1988) showed a 176 percent increase in total iron and a 255 percent increase in ferric iron in the substantia nigra; no changes were observed in the cortex, hippocampus, putamen, or globus pallidus.

Alzheimer's Disease

Iron dysfunction has long been suspected in Alzheimer's disease. Iron is a significant component of senile plaques, and iron encrustation of blood vessels in the brains of patients with Alzheimer's disease is a common observation (Connor, 1992). Iron levels in the hippocampus, amygdala, nucleus basalis of Meynert (Thompson et al., 1988), and the cerebral cortex (Connor et al., 1992) are elevated in patients with Alzheimer's disease. Analyses of iron transport and storage proteins suggest that iron mobility is decreased in the brains of patients with Alzheimer's disease compared with that in the brains of normal subjects (reviewed in Connor, 1992). Decreased iron mobility would likely be associated with decreased metabolic activity and increased peroxidative damage—both well-established phenomena in the brains of patients with Alzheimer's disease, with no known cause. Recently, an iron-responsive element has been reported on the messenger RNA for the amyloid precursor protein (Tanzi and Hyman, 1991; Zubenko et al., 1992), suggesting that iron is somehow involved in regulating amyloid precursor protein synthesis.

Perhaps equally as important as its function in normal activity is the role of iron in oxidative injury leading to membrane damage and, ultimately, cell death (Halliwell, 1991; Zaleska and Floyd, 1985). A decrease in cell membrane fluidity within the central nervous system is considered part of the pathogenesis of aging, and an increase in free-radical production has been demonstrated in the brain tissues of patients with Alzheimer's disease (reviewed in Halliwell, 1991). Iron is a critical factor in the induction of events leading to lipid peroxidative damage in the brain (Zaleska and Floyd, 1985). The relationship between iron and oxidant stress has led to the hypothesis that in patients with Parkinson's disease, iron may contribute to neuronal cell death and tissue damage, especially in the substantia nigra but also in the caudate putamen (Olanow et al., 1992). Thus, the dual nature of iron dictates that it must be both available to cells and stringently regulated. Imbalance of iron or its regulatory proteins in the brain could result in substantial damage to neurons and glia, leading to neurodegeneration and neurologic dysfunction.

Investigators have found that in comparison with normal aged tissue, the transferrin concentration is consistently lower, ferritin levels are either slightly lower or unchanged, and iron levels are elevated in tissues from individuals with Alzheimer's disease (Connor et al., 1992). These observations suggest the decreased mobility of iron and the increased amount of iron stored per mole of ferritin. Such an increase in iron, even if it is stored in ferritin, could increase the likelihood of iron-induced lipid peroxidative damage.

Perhaps most relevant to Alzheimer's disease and iron metabolism are reports of abnormalities in oxidative metabolism in patients with Alzheimer's disease (Gibson and Peterson, 1981). A correlation between the cellular and regional distributions of transferrin receptors and the levels of cytochrome oxidase activity in the brain underscores the importance of iron and oxidative activity (Morris et al., 1992a,b). A recent report has shown a loss of transferrin receptors in specific regions of the brain in patients with Alzheimer's disease, including the hippocampus—an area where mitochondrial enzymes and metabolic activity are decreased in patients with Alzheimer's disease (Gibson and Peterson, 1981; Kalaria et al., 1992). In addition, cholinergic neurotransmission, a well-known defect in patients with Alzheimer's disease, is highly susceptible to impaired oxidative metabolism (Blass and Gibson, 1991; Gibson and Peterson, 1981). This latter observation is particularly exciting in relation to a report that transferrin receptor density is relatively high in the nucleus basalis of Meynert (Morris et al., 1989). The demonstration that iron is also involved in the synthesis and degradation of fatty acids and cholesterol in the brain may have direct relevance to a recent report that cholesterol concentrations are lower in brain regions known to undergo the neurodegenerative changes caused by Alzheimer's disease (Mason et al., 1991).

Recently developed free-radical scavengers and specific iron chelators that cross the blood-brain barrier have already been used as palliative agents in central nervous system trauma. Determination of the effectiveness of these agents in treating Alzheimer's disease would augment existing data. An iron chelator (Desferal) has already been used in a study to abate cognitive decline in patients with Alzheimer's disease (McLachlan et al., 1991). Although the study was controversial in design and interpretation (among other concerns, the study was interpreted to suggest that the effect was due to aluminum without considering the effect of iron), the investigative approach involving iron or aluminum and iron chelation is worthy of pursuit.

Iron-regulatory proteins may also be involved in the development of Alzheimer's disease. Under physiologic conditions, aluminum, which has been implicated in the pathogenesis of Alzheimer's disease, can be bound to transferrin and transported (Aschner and Aschner, 1990; Roskams and Connor, 1990). Roskams and Connor (1990) have shown that a transferrin-aluminum complex can bind to the transferrin receptor in the brain with nearly the same affinity as a transferrin-iron complex. These data suggest that aluminum gains access to the brain by utilizing the extant system for iron transport. Aluminum may also bind to ferritin in patients with Alzheimer's disease, diminishing the ability of ferritin to bind and release iron, further leading to oxidative damage (Dedman et al., 1992; Fleming and Joshi, 1987).

Multiple Sclerosis

The key components necessary to regulate iron delivery, storage, and utilization are found in the highest levels within one cell type in the brain: the oligodendrocyte. Oligodendrocytes are responsible for the production and maintenance of myelin, processes that are disrupted in patients with multiple sclerosis (MS), the prototype of demyelinating diseases. The cellular patterns for iron and transferrin are both altered around MS plaques. Iron is found within MS plaques, and transferrin, which normally should be located in oligodendrocytes, is found instead in astrocytes surrounding MS plaques and in demyelinating areas in central pontine myelinolysis (Craelius et al., 1982; Esiri et al., 1976; Gocht and Lohler, 1990). Recent magnetic resonance imaging data showing iron accumulation in specific brain regions of patients with MS indicate a general disruption in iron regulation (Esiri et al., 1976). Other demyelinating diseases, such as Pelizaeus-Merzbacher disease (reduced transferrin levels and appearance of biochemically abnormal transferrin), progressive rubella panencephalitis (iron deposits in cells in centrum ovale), and the demyelination associated with human immunodeficiency virus infection (siderotic microglia in the demyelinated regions) all strongly indicate that iron homeostasis is disrupted at the cellular level in patients with dysmyelinating disorders (Gelman et al., 1992; Jaeken et al., 1984; Koeppen et al., 1988; Valk, 1989).

The physiology of oligodendrocytes, including the mechanism for myelin production and maintenance, is poorly understood. Although the cause and effect (demyelination) of MS are unknown, induction of oxidative damage by iron has been implicated. In relation to dysmyelinating diseases, the iron-rich, lipid-rich myelin tracts could be a prime target for oxidative damage. Indeed, in an animal model of autoimmune demyelination, the clinical and pathologic symptoms associated with experimental autoimmune neuritis can be reduced in the presence of endogenously administered antioxidants (Hartung et al., 1988).

REFERENCES

Aruoma, O.I., A. Bomford, R.J. Polson, and B. Halliwell. 1988. Nontransferrin-bound iron in plasma from hemochromatosis patients: Effect of phlebotomy therapy. Blood 72:1416–1419.

Aschner, M., and J.L. Aschner. 1990. Manganese transport across the blood brain barrier: Relationship to iron homeostasis. Brain Res. Bull. 24:857–860.

Balla, G., H.S. Jacob, J. Balla, et al. 1991. Ferritin: A cytoprotective antioxidant strategem of endothelium. J. Biol. Chem. 267:18148–18153.

Benito, E. 1991. Nutritional factors in colorectal cancer risk. Intern. J. Cancer 49:161–167.

Blass, J.P., and G.E. Gibson. 1991. The role of oxidative abnormalities in the pathophysiology of Alzheimer's disease. Rev. Neurol. 147:513.

Bolann, B.J., and R.J. Ulvik. 1990. On the limited ability of superoxide to release iron from ferritin. Eur. J. Biochem. 193:899–904.

Bothwell, T.H., and R.W. Charlton. 1982. A general approach to the problems of iron deficiency and iron overload in the population at large. Pp. 54–67 in Seminars in Hematology, P.A. Miescher and F.R. Jaffe, eds. New York: Grune & Stratton, Inc.

Connor, J.R. 1992. Proteins of iron regulation in the brain in Alzheimer's disease. Pp. 365–393 in Iron and Human Disease, R.B. Lauffer, ed. Ann Arbor, Mich.: CRC Press.

Connor, J.R., B.S. Snyder, J.L. Beard, R.E. Fine, and E.J. Mufson. 1992. The regional distribution of iron and iron regulatory proteins in the brain in aging and Alzheimer's disease. J. Neurosci. Res. 31:327.

Cozzi, A., P. Santambrogio, S. Levi, and P. Arosio. 1990. Iron detoxifying activity of ferritin: Effects of H and I human apoferritins on lipid peroxidation in vitro. FEBS Lett. 177:119–122.

Craelius, W., M.W. Migdal, C.P. Luessenhop, A. Sugar, and I. Mihalakis. 1982. Iron deposits surrounding multiple sclerosis plaques. Arch. Pathol. Lab. Med. 106:397–399.

Crighton, R.R., F. Roman, and F. Roaldn. 1980. Iron mobilization from ferritin by chelating agents. J. Inorg. Biochem. 13:305–316.

Dedman, D.J., A. Treffry, J.M. Candy, G.A. Taylor, C.M. Morris, C.A. Bloxham, R.H. Perry, J.A. Edwardson, and P.M. Harrison. 1992. Iron and aluminum in relation to brain ferritin in normal individuals and Alzheimer's disease and chronic renal-dialysis patients. Biochem. J. 287:509–514.

Drayer, B., P. Burger, B. Horwitz, D. Dawson, and J. Cain. 1987. Reduced signal intensity on MR images of thalamus and putamen in MS. Am. J. Neuroradiol. 8:413–419.

Esiri, M.M., C.R. Taylor, and D.Y. Mason. 1976. Applications of an immunoperoxidase method to a study of the central nervous system: Preliminary findings in a study of human formalin-fixed material. Neuropathol. Appl. Neurobiol. 2:233–246.

Evans, P.J., R. Evans, I.Z. Kovar, A.F. Holton, and B. Halliwell. 1992. Bleomycin-detectable iron in the plasma of premature and full-term neonates. FEBS Lett. 303:210–212.

Fleming, J., and J.G. Joshi. 1987. Ferritin: Isolation of aluminum-ferritin complex from brain. Proc. Natl. Acad. Sci. USA 84:7866.

Floyd, R.A. 1983. Direct demonstration that ferrous iron complexes of di- and triphosphate nucleotides catalyze hydroxyl free radical formation from hydrogen peroxide. Arch. Biochem. Biophys. 225:263–270.

Foerder, C.A., A.A. Tobin, G.B. McDonald, and R.A. Zager. 1992. Bleomycin-detectable iron in plasma of bone-marrow transplantation patients—its correlation with liver injury. Transplantation 54:1120–1123.

Friedman, G.D., and H.K. Ury. 1980. Initial screening for carcinogenicity of commonly used drugs. J. Natl. Cancer Inst. 65:723–733.

Friedman, G.D., and H.K. Ury. 1983. Screening for possible drug carcinogenicity: Second report of findings. J. Natl. Cancer Inst. 71:1165–1175.

Gelman, B.B., M.S. Rodriguz-Wolf, and J. Wen. 1992. Siderotic cerebral macrophages in the acquired immunodeficiency syndrome. Arch. Pathol. Lab. Med. 116:509.

Gibson, G.E., and C.P. Peterson. 1981. Aging decreases oxidative metabolism and the release and synthesis of acetylcholine. J. Neurochem. 37:978.

Gocht, A., and J. Lohler. 1990. Changes in glial cell markers in recent and old demyelinated lesions in central pontine myelinolysis. Acta Neuropathol. 80:46–58.

Gordeuk, V.R., and G.M. Brittenham. 1992. Bleomycin-reactive iron in patients with acute non-lymphocytic leukemia. FEBS Lett. 308:4–6.

Groenwald, G., M.L. Langenhoven, M.J.C. Beyers, J.P. DuPlessis, J.J. Ferriera, and S.J. van Reusbary. 1981. Nutrient intakes among rural Tanskeins at risk for esophageal cancer. SA Mediese Tydskraf 964–967.

Gutteridge, J.M.C. 1986. Antioxidant properties of the proteins caeruloplasmin, albumin and transerrin, a study of their activity in serum and synovial fluid from patients with rheumatoid arthritis. Biochem. Biophys. Acta 869:119–127.

Gutteridge, J.M.C. 1987. The antioxidant activity of haptoglobin towards haemoglobin-stimulated lipid peroxidation. Bichem. Biophys. Acta 917:219–223.

Gutteridge, J.M.C. 1992. Ferrous ions detected in cerebrospinal fluid by using bleomycin and DNA damage. Clin. Sci. 82:315–320.

Gutteridge, J.M.C., R. Richmond, and B. Halliwell. 1980. Oxygen free-radicals and lipid peroxidation: Inhibition by the protein caeruloplasmin. FEBS Lett. 112:269–272.

Gutteridge, J.M.C., S.K. Patterson, A.W. Segal, and B. Halliwell. 1981. Inhibition of lipid peroxidation by the iron-binding protein lactoferrin. Biochem. J. 199:259–261.

Gutteridge, J.M.C., B. Halliwell, A. Treffry, P.M. Harrison, and D. Blake. 1983. Effect of ferritin fractions with different iron loading on lipid peroxidation. Biochem. J. 209:557–560.

Hallgren, B., and P. Sourander. 1958. The effect of age on the nonhaemin iron in the human brain. J. Neurochem. 3:41–51.

Halliwell, B. 1987. Oxidants and human disease: Some new concepts. FASEB J. 1:358–364.

Halliwell, B. 1991. Reactive oxygen species in living systems: Source, biochemistry, and role of human disease. Am. J. Med. 91(Suppl. 3c):14S–22S.

Halliwell, B., and J.M.C. Gutteridge. 1990. Role of free radicals and catalytic metal ions in human disease: An overview. Methods Enzymol. 186:1–85.

Harrison, P.M., T.G. Hoy, I.G. Macara, and R.J. Hoare. 1974. Ferritin iron uptake and release: Structure-function relationships. Biochem. J. 143:445–451.

Hartung, H.P., B. Schafer, K. Heininger, and K.V. Toyka. 1988. Suppression of experimental autoimmune neuritis by the oxygen radical scavenger superoxide dismutase and catalase. Ann. Neurol. 23:453–460.

Hoff, G., I.E. Molen, K. Trygg, W. Frolich, J. Sauer, et al. 1986. Epidemiology of polyps in the rectum and sigmoid colon. Scand. J. Gastroenterol. 21:199–204.

Jaeken, J., H.G. van Eijk, C. Van der Heul, and I. Corbeel. 1984. Folic acid-deficient serum and cerebrospinal fluid transferrin in a newly recognized genetic disorder. Clin. Chim. Acta 144:245–247.

Kalaria, R.N., S.M. Sromek, I. Grahovac, and S.I. Harik. 1992. Transferrin receptors of rat and human brain and cerebral microvessels and their status in Alzheimer's disease. Brain Res. 585:87–93.

Karlsson, M., E. Ikkala, A. Reunanen, H. Takkunen, E. Vuori, and J. Makinen. 1988. Prevalence of hemochromatosis in Finland. Acta Med. Scand. 224:385–390.

Koeppen, A.H., K.D. Barron, C.K. Csiza, and E.A. Greenfield. 1988. Comparative immunocytochemistry of Palizaeus-Merzbacher disease, the jimpy, mouse and the myelin-deficient rat. J. Neurol. Sci. 84:315–327.

Kuzuya, M., M. Naito, K. Yamada, et al. 1990. Involvement of intracellular iron in the toxicity of oxidized low density lipoprotein to cultured endothelial cells. Biochem. Int. 22:567–573.

Mason, R.P., I. Shajenko, T.E. Chambers, H.J. Grazioso, W.J. Shoemaker, and L.G. Herbette. 1991. Biochemical and structural analysis of lipid membranes from temporal gyrus and cerebellum of Alzheimer's diseased brains. Biophys. J. 59:592.

McLachlan, D.R.C., A.J. Dalton, T.P.A. Kruck, M.Y. Bell, W.L. Smith, W. Kalow, and D.F. Andrews. 1991. Intramuscular desferrioxamine in patients with Alzheimer's disease. Lancet 337:1304.

Minetti, M., T. Forte, M. Soriani, et al. 1992. Iron-induced ascorbate oxidation in plasma as monitored by ascorbate free radical formation. No spin-trapping evidence for the hydroxyl radical in iron-overloaded plasma. Biochem J. 282:459–465.

Moison, R.M.W., J.J.S. Palinckx, M. Roest, E. Houdkamp, and H.M. Berger. 1993. Induction of lipid peroxidation of pulmonary surfactant by plasma of preterm babies. Lancet 341:79–82.

Monteiro, H.P., and C.C. Winterbourn. 1988. The superoxide-dependent transfer of iron from ferritin to transferrin and lactoferrin. Biochem. J. 256:923–928.

Morris, C.M., J.M. Candy, A.E. Oakley, G.A. Taylor, S. Mountfort, H. Bishop, M.K. Ward, C.A. Bloxham, and J.A. Edwardson. 1989. Comparison of the regional distribution of transferrin receptors and aluminum in the forebrain of chronic renal dialysis patients. J. Neurol. Sci. 94:295–306.

Morris, C.M., J.M. Candy, C.A. Bloxham, and J.A. Edwardson. 1992a. Distribution of transferrin receptors in relation to cytochrome oxidase activity in the human spinal cord, lower brainstem and cerebellum. J. Neurol. Sci. 111:158–172.

Morris, C.M., J.M. Candy, A.E. Oakley, C.A. Bloxham, and J.A. Edwardson. 1992b. Histochemical distribution of non-haem iron in the human brain. Acta Anat. 144:235–257.

Olanow, C.W., D. Marsden, D. Perl, and G. Cohen, eds. 1992. Iron and oxidative stress in Parkinson's disease. Ann. Neurol. 32:Suppl.

Pillay, T.S., and M.W. Makgoba. 1992. Bleomycin-reactive iron in patients with acute non-lymphocytic leukemia. FEBS Lett. 308:4–6.

Puppo, A., and B. Halliwell. 1988. Formation of hydroxyl radicals from hydrogen peroxide in the presence of iron. Is haemoglobin a biological Fenton reagent? Biochem. J. 249:185–190.

Reif, D.W. 1992. Ferritin as a souce of iron for oxidative damage. Free Radical Biol. Med. 12:417–427.

Rimm, E., A. Ascherio, M.J. Stampfer, G.A. Colditz, E. Giovannucci, and W.C. Willett. 1993. Dietary iron intake and risk of coronary disease among men. Circulation 87:692 abstract P22.

Roskams, A.J., and J.R. Connor. 1990. Aluminum access to the brain: A possible role for the transferrin receptor. Proc. Natl. Acad. Sci. USA 87:9024.

Salonen, J.T., K. Nyyssönen, H. Korpela, J. Tuomilehto, and S.R. Seppänen. 1992. High stored iron levels are associated with excess risk of myocardial infarction. Circulation 86:803–811.

Samokyszyn, V.M., D.M. Miller, D.W. Reif, and S.D. Aust. 1989. Inhibition of superoxide and ferritin-dependent lipid peroxidation by ceruloplasmin. J. Biol. Chem. 264:21–26.

Samokyszyn, V.M., D.W. Reif, D.M. Miller, and S.D. Aust. 1991. Effects of ceruloplasmin on superoxide-dependent iron release from ferritin and lipid peroxidation. Free Radical Res. Commun. 12-13:153–159.

Selby, J.V., and G.D. Friedman. 1988. Epidemiologic evidence of an association between body iron stores and risk of cancer. Int. J. Cancer 41:677–682.

Siegers, C.P., D. Bumann, G. Baretton, and M. Younes. 1988. Dietary iron enhances the tumor rate in dimethylhydrazine-induced colon carcinogenesis in mice. Cancer Lett. 41:251–256.

Siegers, C.P., D. Bumman, H.D. Trepkau, B. Schadwinkel, and G. Barretton. 1992. Influence of dietary iron overload on cell proliferation and intestinal tumorigenesis in mice. Cancer Lett. 65:245–249.

Smith, C., M.J., Mitchinson, O.I. Aruoma, and B. Halliwell. 1992. Stimulation of lipid peroxidation and hydroxyl-radical generation by the contents of human atheroxelerotic lesions. Biochem. J. 286:901–905.

Sofic, E., P. Riederer, H. Heinsen, H. Beckmann, G.P. Reynolds, G. Hebenstreit, and M.B. Youdim. 1988. Increased iron(III) and total iron content in postmortem substantia nigra of Parkinsonian brain. J. Neural Trans. 74:199–205.

Steinberg, D., S. Parthasarathy, T.E. Carew, J.C. Khoo, and J.L. Witztum. 1989. Beyond cholesterol. N. Engl. J. Med. 320:915–924.

Stevens, R.G., R.P. Beasley, and B.S. Blumberg. 1986. Iron-binding proteins and risk of cancer in Taiwan. JNCI 76:605–610.

Stevens, R.G., D.Y. Jones, M.S. Micozzi, and P.R. Taylor. 1988. Body iron stores and the risk of cancer. N. Engl. J. Med. 319:1047–1052.

Swaiman, K.F. 1991. Hallervorden-Spatz syndrome and brain iron metabolism. Arch. Neurol. 48:1285–1293.

Tanzi, R.E., and B.T. Hyman. 1991. Alzheimer's mutation (letter). Nature 350:564.

Thomas, C.E., I.A. Morehouse, and S.D. Aust. 1985. Ferritin and superoxide-dependent lipid peroxidation. J. Biol. Chem. 260:3275–3280.

Thompson, C.M., W.R. Marksberry, W.D. Ehmann, Y.Y. Mao, and D.E. Vance. 1988. Regional brain trace-element studies in Alzheimer's disease. Neurotoxicology 9:1.

Thompson, H.J., K. Kennedy, M. Witt, and J. Juzefyk. 1991. Effect of dietary iron deficiency or excess on the induction of mammary carcinogenesis by 1-methyl-1-nitrosourea. Carcinogenesis 12:111–114.

Valk, J. 1989. Magnetic Resonance of Myelin, Myelination and Myelin Disorders. New York: Springer-Verlag.

Van der Kraaij, A.M.M., I.J. Mostert, H.G. Van Eijk, and J.F. Koster. 1988. Iron-load increases the susceptibility of rat hearts to oxygen reperfusion damage: Protection by the antioxidant (+)-cyanidanol-3 and deferoxamine. Circulation 78:442–449.

Vitale, J.P., S.A. Broitman, E. Vavrousek-Jakuba, P.W. Rodday, and L.S. Gottlieb. 1977. The effects of iron deficiency and the quality and quantity of fat on chemically induced cancer. Adv. Exp. Med. Biol. 91:229–242.

Williams, R.F., J.I. Zweier, and J.T. Flaherty. 1991. Treatment with deferoxamine during ischemia improves functional and metabolic recovery and reduces reperfusion-induced oxygen radical generation in rabbit hearts. Circulation 83:1006–1014.

Yoshigi, K., D. Nakae, Y. Mizumoto, K. Horiguchi, et al. 1992. Inhibitory effect of dietary iron deficiency on inductions of putative preneoplastic lesions as well as 8-hydroxy-deoxyguanosine in DNA and lipid peroxidation in the livers of rats caused by exposure to a choline-deficient L-amino acid defined diet. Carcinogenesis 13(7):1227–1233.

Zaleska, M.M., and R. Floyd. 1985. Regional lipid peroxidation in rat brain in vitro: Possible role of endogenous iron. Neurochem. Res. 10:397.

Zubenko, G.S., J. Farr, J.S. Stiffer, H.B. Hughes, and B.B. Kaplan. 1992. Clinically silent mutation in the putative iron-response element in exon 17 of the ß-amyloid precursor protein gene. J. Neuropathol. Exp. Neurol. 51(4):459–466.

D

Dietary Iron: Trends in the Iron Content of Foods, Use of Supplemental Iron, and the Framework for Regulation of Iron in the Diet

TRENDS IN THE IRON CONTENT OF FOODS AND CONSUMPTION FROM DIET AND THE USE OF SUPPLEMENTS

Dietary Consumption Patterns

The foods that contribute most to dietary iron are grain products and meat, poultry, and fish (LSRO, 1989). As shown in Figure D-1, the contribution from grain products has increased since estimates of specific food contributions to the food supply were first made in 1909. The reasons for the increases are enrichment of white flour with iron and other nutrients (since World War II) and the increased use of iron-fortified cereal products.

Data from several sources indicate that the levels of iron in the diets of infants and toddlers increased during the 1970s and 1980s. Although data from the Total Diet Study, which provided reporting on the chemical analyses of typical diets, showed no change from 1974 to 1982 (Table D-1) (Pennington et al., 1984), the average iron intakes from four national surveys conducted from 1971 to 1986 indicate increases for children 1–2 and 3–5 years of age (Table D-2) (LSRO, 1989).

For adult women, no change in the iron contents of typical diets (Table D-1) or intakes (Table D-2) during the 1970s and 1980s was observed.

Infant Cereals

Iron preparations that are soluble in water or in dilute acid (such as in the stomach) are generally of high bioavailability, whereas forms of iron that are insoluble in water or dilute acid solutions are of low bioavailability (Hurrell, 1992). Examples of iron salts that are freely soluble both in water and in dilute acid are ferrous sulfate, ferrous ascorbate, ferrous gluconate, and ferric ammonium citrate. Examples of salts that are poorly soluble in water but soluble in

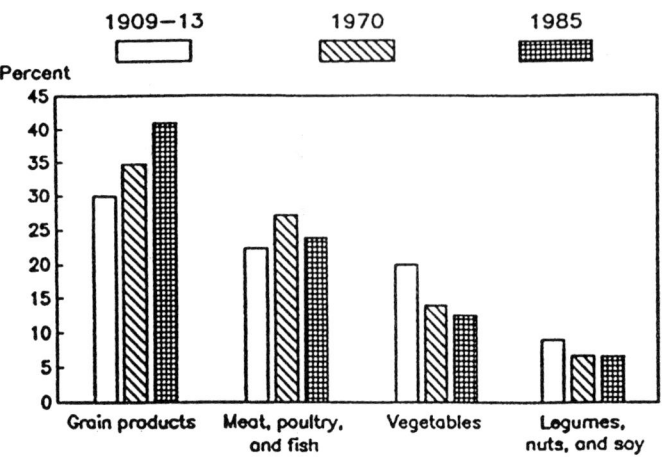

FIGURE D-1 Major food sources of iron in the food supply. SOURCE: LSRO (1989).

dilute acids are ferrous fumarate, ferrous succinate, and ferric saccharate. Many of the iron preparations commonly used for food fortification are poorly soluble in water and poorly soluble in dilute acid (e.g., ferric pyrophosphate and ferric orthophosphate, which were used in the past, and elemental iron powders of intermediate particle size).

In the presence of oxygen, water-soluble forms of iron react with various components of food to produce oxidative rancidity. Such forms of iron can be used to fortify foods that can be packaged to limit prolonged contact with oxygen (e.g., infant formulas). Dry cereals packaged in cardboard boxes (including cereals specifically marketed for infants) permit exchange of air between package contents and the environment, and it is therefore not feasible to fortify them with ferrous sulfate or with most other iron salts known to have good bioavailability (Coccodrilli et al., 1976; Hurrell, 1984). In the United States, most dry infant cereals are fortified with a metallic iron powder, specifically, electrolytic iron.

The bioavailabilities of metallic iron powders are closely related to particle size and solubility (Björn-Rasmussen et al., 1977). Metallic iron powders of extremely small particle size are readily soluble in dilute acid (Björn-Rasmussen et al., 1977) and have good bioavailability (Björn-Rasmussen et al., 1977; Rios et al., 1975). Unfortunately, the greater the solubility (and, presumably, the greater the bioavailability) of a metallic iron powder, the greater its chemical reactivity and the less suitable it is for food fortification. Circumstantial evidence has led several authors to conclude that electrolytic iron powder of the

TABLE D-1 Iron Levels in Diets of Adult Males, Infants, and Toddlers

Diet and Year	No. of Collections	Iron Level (mg/day) Mean	Standard Deviation
Adult diets			
1974	30	20.0^{ab}	3.0
1975	20	18.0^{b}	3.1
1976	20	18.2^{ab}	3.1
1977	25	18.3^{ab}	5.8
1978	20	17.9^{b}	4.1
1979	20	18.3^{ab}	4.2
1980	20	21.0^{a}	5.1
1981–82	27	18.4^{ab}	3.2
Infant diets			
1975	10	7.4^{a}	5.7
1976	10	7.3^{a}	4.0
1977	12	6.8^{a}	3.6
1978	10	4.7^{a}	2.1
1979	10	9.6^{a}	10.3
1980	10	10.2^{a}	4.8
1981–82	13	9.5^{a}	6.3
Toddler diets			
1975	10	11.1^{a}	3.8
1975	10	10.1^{a}	3.2
1977	12	8.5^{a}	2.6
1978	10	7.7^{a}	2.3
1979	10	11.9^{a}	11.5
1980	10	9.1^{a}	12.0
1981–1982	13	9.0^{a}	1.7

NOTE: Mean values within each diet category with the same superscript are not significantly different. Adult diets are based on 2,850 kcal/day. Infant (6 months) diets are based on 880 kcal/day. Toddler (2 years) diets are based on 1,300 kcal/day.

SOURCE: Pennington et al. (1984).

TABLE D-2 Mean Iron Intake by Sex and Age in 1 day from NHANES I and II, NFCS, and CSFII

	Iron Intake (mg)[a]							
	NHANES I 1971–1974		NFCS 1977–1978		NHANES II 1976–1980		CSFII 1985–1986	
Sex and Age (yr)	Mean	SEM	Mean	SEM	Mean	SEM	Mean	SEM
Both sexes								
1–2	7.35	0.16	8.1	0.16	8.57	0.13	10.2	0.51
3–5	8.58	0.11	9.5	0.12	10.02	0.09	11.0	0.34
6–11	10.81	0.17	12.2	0.12	12.34	0.31	—	—
Male								
12–15	14.13	0.42	15.6	0.20	16.01	0.45	—	—
16–19	16.70	0.51	16.9	0.26	18.15	0.60	—	—
20–29[b]	16.55	0.40	16.2	0.23	17.59	0.45	16.7	0.79
30–39[b]	16.54	0.48	15.9	0.21	16.48	0.49	15.6	0.70
40–49[b]	15.26	0.42	16.1	0.24	16.58	0.53	15.6	0.81
50–59	13.85	0.38	15.9	0.23	15.21	0.43	—	—
60–69	13.08	0.18	14.9	0.25	14.73	0.20	—	—
70+[c]	11.68	0.16	14.2	0.28	13.24	0.29	—	—
Female								
12–15	10.44	0.28	11.9	0.21	10.71	0.32	—	—
16–19[b]	9.54	0.30	11.2	0.20	10.04	0.34	—	—
20–29[b]	10.06	0.13	10.7	0.17	10.67	0.23	11.1	0.27
30–39[b]	10.36	0.14	11.1	0.15	11.08	0.31	11.1	0.26
40–49	10.40	0.18	11.0	0.14	11.10	0.34	10.6	0.22
50–59	10.15	0.28	11.5	0.17	10.30	0.30	—	—
60–69	9.53	0.14	11.0	0.15	10.53	0.13	—	—
70+[c]	8.63	0.13	10.4	0.16	10.18	0.22	—	—

[a] SEM is standard error of the mean, NHANES I and II are the first and second national Health and Nutrition Examination Surveys, NFCS is the Nationwide Food Consumption Survey, and CSFII is the Continuing Survey of Food Intakes of Individuals.
[b] Data from CSFII are for 1985 only.
[c] Ages 70–74 years only for NHANES I and NHANES II.

SOURCE: LSRO (1989).

particle size currently used to fortify infant cereals in the United States is of low bioavailability (Fomon, 1987; Hurrell, 1984; Hurrell et al., 1989). A similar conclusion was reached by Hallberg et al. (1986) for another metallic iron powder with similar solubility.

Infant cereals fortified with electrolytic iron powder are among the first breakfast items introduced into the infant's diet. A large study carried out in Chile (Walter et al., 1993) demonstrated that feeding of infant cereal fortified with electrolytic iron powder can exert a favorable effect on iron nutritional status; at an intake level of 26–30 g of iron per day, fortified cereal was slightly but not significantly less effective in preventing iron deficiency anemia than iron-fortified infant formula. Whether the much lower intakes of cereal likely to be fed to infants in the United States (mean consumption for 73 percent of 6- to 12-month-old infants was 19 g/day in one infant nutrition survey [Gerber Products Company, 1989]) would contribute substantially to meeting infants' needs for absorbed iron is unknown. Findings from a recent, as yet unpublished Canadian study indicate that fortified cereal is effective in meeting the iron needs of infants; intake of cereal was about 33 g/day for 6- to 12-month-old infants (Beaton et al., in press).

Potential Role of Meat in Meeting Infants' Need for Absorbed Iron

The potential role of meat in the diets of older infants and preschool-age children is based on its contribution of heme iron and on the enhancing effect of meat on absorption of non-heme iron. Studies of iron absorption from meals indicate that adults with moderate iron stores (500 mg) generally absorb less than 5 percent of dietary non-heme iron and about 25 percent of dietary heme iron (Monsen et al., 1978). Although heme iron provides only 5 to 10 percent of the iron in the adult Western diet, it accounts for more than one-third of the absorbed iron (Cook, 1983).

The iron content of cooked beef generally ranges from 2.0 to 3.0 mg/100 g (Pennington, 1989). Assuming that heme iron makes up about 70 percent of the iron present in cooked beef (the heme content of raw beef has been reported by Hazell [1982] to be 78 percent of total iron and by Schricker and colleagues [1982] to be 62 percent of total iron; little heme iron is likely to be destroyed by cooking), 100 g of cooked beef provides about 1.75 mg of heme iron. Thus, with 25 percent absorption, consumption of 30 g of cooked beef per day by an infant or preschool-age child might result in absorption of 0.13 mg of heme iron per day (1.75 mg/100 g × 30 g × 0.25). In addition, the presence of meat in the meal would enhance absorption of non-heme iron from meat and other foods in the meal. The effect of animal tissue protein on absorption of non-heme iron is dose related, with 1 g of meat exerting about the same enhancing effect as 1 mg of ascorbic acid (Cook, 1983). Therefore, an intake of 30 g of meat would be expected to exert a major effect on total iron absorption.

Use of Supplemental Iron Products

Supplement use has been assessed by three national surveys conducted between 1971 and 1986. The first National Health and Nutrition Examination Survey (NHANES I), conducted from 1971 to 1974, found that 23 percent of U.S. adults took supplements daily (Block et al., 1988). A special survey conducted by the U.S. Food and Drug Administration (FDA) in 1980 found that about 40 percent of adults reported using a vitamin or mineral product regularly (Stewart et al., 1985). In the 1986 National Health Interview Survey, investigators conducted detailed interviews and found that 36 percent of adults took a vitamin-mineral supplement (Moss et al., 1989). The survey found that 24.5 percent of women 18–44 years of age reported using a supplement containing iron, and the median average daily intake of iron was 100 percent of the Recommended Dietary Allowance (RDA). The estimated 90th percentile of intake from supplements was 247 percent of the RDA, and the 95th percentile of intake was 345 percent of the RDA. In further analysis of this survey, Looker and colleagues (1990) reported that iron supplement use among women 18 to 44 years of age was highest for whites (26 percent) and lower for blacks (15 percent) and Hispanics (16 percent).

REGULATORY FRAMEWORK FOR IRON ENRICHMENT AND FORTIFICATION

Iron in various forms is used for both enrichment and fortification of food products. FDA currently allows added iron compounds to be used as a nutrient or flavoring in food products. The FDA currently certifies 16 types of iron for use as a nutrient or flavor (Table D-3).

Current food industry practice for iron fortification and enrichment of food varies. By regulation (21 CFR §107.100), iron-fortified infant formula must contain between 0.15 and 3.0 mg of iron per 100 kcal of formula. Infant cereals and foods generally use electrolytic iron (dry cereals) and ferrous sulfate (jarred, ready-to-eat [RTE] infant cereals) and provide approximately 45 percent of the U.S. Recommended Daily Allowance (U.S. RDA) for infants per serving.

RTE breakfast cereals are generally fortified with reduced iron, the particle size of which is controlled. Many products also contain supplemental ascorbic acid (vitamin C). RTE breakfast cereals generally supply 10 to 100 percent of the U.S. RDA for iron per serving, but most, on the average, contain between 25 and 45 percent of the U.S. RDA for iron per serving. Forty-five percent of the U.S. RDA is the minimum amount of iron per serving required for an RTE breakfast cereal to be approved for use with the Special Supplemental Food Program for Women, Infants, and Children (WIC).

TABLE D-3 Iron Compounds Certified for Use in Foods

Compound	21 CFR §[a]	Use[b]
Ferric:		
Ammonium citrate	184.1296	N
Chloride	184.1297	F, other
Citrate	184.1298	N
Phosphate	182.5301/184.1301	N
Pyrophosphate	182.5304/184.1304	N
Sulfate	184.1307	F
Sodium pyrophosphate	182.5306	DS
Ferrous:		
Ascorbate	184.1307a	N
Carbonate	184.1307b	N
Citrate	184.1307c	N
Fumarate	184.1307d	N
Gluconate	182.5308/184.1308	N
Lactate	182.5311/184.1311	N
Sulfate	182.5315/184.1315	N
Reduced iron (elemental iron; electrolytic or carbonyl)	182.5375/184.1375	N
Iron-choline citrate complex	172.370	N, DS

[a] Citations from Section 182 are generally recognized as safe (GRAS) for use in dietary supplements (pills); citations from Section 184 are GRAS and are affirmed for use in foods.
[b] DS, dietary supplement; F, flavor; N, nutrient.

SOURCE: 21 CFR (1992). (Additional information was obtained from personal commun-ication with George Pauli, Center for Food Safety and Applied Nutrition, FDA, May 1993.)

Food companies began to enrich milled grain products in the late 1940s. Enrichment of flour and other grain products with iron (and thiamin, riboflavin, and niacin) began as a mechanism to reduce diseases and conditions of nutrient deficiency. Over the years, this public intervention has been remarkably effective and efficient for enhancing the nutrient quality of the food supply. The most common types of iron used to fortify flour and other grain products are hydrogen-reduced elemental iron (cereals, rice, flours) and ferrous sulfate (pasta).

At present, a significant amount of research is being conducted to evaluate ways to increase iron intake. Many new iron compounds for use in fortification and enrichment are being evaluated. The problem is that the bioavailability of iron compounds is generally inversely related to their reactivities in foods. Thus, the most readily available forms tend to discolor food and catalyze fat oxidation. Other approaches involve the addition of substances to foods that increase iron absorption from the gut (i.e., ascorbic acid or meat). More research is being conducted on the precise component of meat that influences iron absorption. In projects in developing countries, iron-EDTA is being evaluated as a vehicle for delivering iron. In Sweden, ferrous ammonium phosphate is being studied for use in foods.

New food labeling regulations required by the Nutrition Labeling and Education Act of 1990 (P.L. 101-535) have implications for iron-enriched and fortified food products. The law and implementing regulations change both the legal status and the expression of iron on the food label. Past regulations required a listing of iron content only if it was added to a food or if a claim was made about its content. New serving sizes for RTE breakfast cereals may require additional consumer education to inform consumers about the amount of iron in a serving and may force some product reformulation for the cereals to continue to be certified for use with the WIC program.

REFERENCES

Beaton, G.H, P. Tanaka, S. Zlotkin, G.H. Anderson, I.A. Menon, and D.L. Young. In press. Efficacy of Iron Fortification of Infant Cereals. Final report to the National Health Research Development Program, Canada, Toronto, Ontario, Canada.

Björn-Rasmussen, E., L. Hallberg, and L. Rossander. 1977. Absorption of "fortification" iron: Bioavailability in man of different samples of reduced Fe, and prediction of the effects of Fe fortification. Br. J. Nutr. 37:175–188.

Block, G., C. Cox, J. Madans, G.B. Schreiber, L. Licitra, and N. Melia. 1988. Vitamin supplement use by demographic characteristics. Am. J. Epidemiol. 127:297–309.

Coccodrilli, G.D., Jr., G.H. Reussner, and R. Thiessen, Jr. 1976. Relative biological value of iron supplements in processed food products. J. Agric. Food Chem. 24:351–353.

Cook, J.D. 1983. Determinants of nonheme iron absorption in man. Food Technol. (October):124–126.

Fomon, S.J. 1987. Bioavailability of supplemental iron in commercially prepared dry infant cereals. J. Pediatr. 110:660–661.

Gerber Products Company. 1989. Infant Nutrition Survey. Fremont, Mich.: Gerber Products Company.

Hallberg, L., M. Brune, and L. Rossander. 1986. Low bioavailability of carbonyl iron in man: Studies on iron fortification of wheat flour. Am J. Clin. Nutr. 43:59–67.

Hazell, T. 1982. Iron and zinc compounds in the muscle meats of beef, lamb, pork and chicken. J. Sci. Food Agric. 33:1049–1056.

Hurrell, R.F. 1984. Bioavailability of different iron compounds used to fortify formulas and cereals: Technological problems. Pp. 147–148 in Iron Nutrition in Infancy and Childhood, A. Stekel, ed. New York: Raven Press.

Hurrell, R.F. 1992. Prospects for improving the iron fortification of foods. Pp. 193–208 in Nutritional Anemias, S.J. Fomon and S.H. Zlotkin, eds. New York: Raven Press.

Hurrell, R.F., D.E. Furniss, J. Burr, P. Whittaker, S.R. Lynch, and J.D. Cook. 1989. Iron fortification in infant cereals: A proposal for the use of ferrous fumarate or ferrous succinate. Am. J. Clin. Nutr. 49:1274–1282.

Looker, A.C., C.M. Loria, M.A. McDowell, and C.L. Johnson. 1990. Dietary habits of blacks and other ethnic minorities in the U.S. with special references to iron status. Pp. 15–23 in Functional Significance of Iron Deficiency, C.O. Enwonwu, ed. Nashville: Meharry Medical College.

LSRO (Life Sciences Research Office). 1989. Nutrition Monitoring in the United States—An Update Report on Nutrition Monitoring. DHHS Publication No. (PHS) 89-1255. Public Health Service. Washington, D.C.: U.S. Government Printing Office.

Monsen, E.R., L. Hallberg, M. Layrisse, D.M. Hegsted, J.D. Cook, W. Mertz, and C.A. Finch. 1978. Estimation of available dietary iron. Am. J. Clin. Nutr. 31:134–141.

Moss, A.J., A.S. Levy, I. Kim, and Y.K. Park. 1989. Use of vitamin and mineral supplements in the United States: current users, types of products, and nutrients. Advance Data from Vital and Health Statistics. 174.

Pennington, J.A.T. 1989. Bowes and Church's Food Values of Portions Commonly Used, 15th ed. New York: Harper & Row.

Pennington, J.A.T., D.C. Wilson, R.F. Newell, et al. 1984. Selected minerals in foods surveys, 1974 to 1981/82. J. Am. Diet. Assoc. 84:771–782.

Rios, E., R.E. Hunter, J.D. Cook, N.J. Smith, and C.A. Finch. 1975. The absorption of iron as supplements in infant cereal and infant formula. Pediatrics 55:686–693.

Schricker, B.R., D.D. Miller, and J.R. Stouffer. 1982. Measurement and content of nonheme and total iron in muscle. J. Food Sci. 47:740–743.

Stewart, M.L., J.T. McDonald, A.S. Levy, R.E. Schucker, and D.P. Henderson. 1985. Vitamin and mineral supplement use: A telephone survey of adults in the United States. J. Am. Diet. Assoc. 85:1585–1590.

Walter, T., P.R. Dallman, F. Pizarro, L. Veloso, G. Peña, S. Bartholmey, E. Hertrampf, M. Olivares, A. Letelier, and M. Arredondo. 1993. Effectiveness of iron-fortified infant cereal in prevention of iron deficiency anemia. Pediatrics 91:976–982.

E

Committee and Staff Biographies

COMMITTEE

DORIS HOWES CALLOWAY (*Chair*) is Professor Emerita of Nutrition, Department of Nutrition, University of California at Berkeley. She has also served as Provost of the University of California at Berkeley. A member of the Institute of Medicine, Dr. Calloway has served on the Food and Nutrition Board (FNB) and was a member of the FNB Committee to Revise the 10th Edition of the Recommended Dietary Allowances. She is an active international consultant on human nutrition and food issues and is a recipient of the Elvehjem Award of the American Institute of Nutrition. She is a member and past president of the American Institute of Nutrition. Dr. Calloway holds a B.S. from the Ohio State University and a Ph.D. from the University of Chicago.

JOHN L. BEARD is a Professor in the Departments of Nutrition and Biobehavioral Health in the College of Health and Human Development, The Pennsylvania State University, University Park. Dr. Beard is an ad hoc reviewer for the *Journal of Nutrition, Clinical Nutrition, Nutrition Today,* the *American Journal of Clinical Nutrition,* and has served on the U.S.Department of Agriculture Competitive Grants Program review panel. He is a member of the American Institute of Nutrition, the American Society for Clinical Nutrition, the American College of Sports Medicine, and the Center for the Study of Child and Adolescent Development. Dr. Beard holds a B.S. from the Stevens Institute of Technology, Hoboken, New Jersey; an M.S. from the University of California at Santa Cruz; and a Ph.D. from Cornell University.

GEORGE H. BEATON (consultant) is Professor of Nutritional Sciences in the Faculty of Medicine, University of Toronto, Ontario, Canada. He has served as chair of the Department of Nutritional Sciences and head of the earlier Department of Nutrition, as acting director of the School of Hygiene (Public Health), and as acting dean of the Faculty of Food Sciences in that university. Dr. Beaton has worked with several National Academy of Sciences committees and has had extensive imvolvement with the World Health Organization and other United Nations agencies. He received the Borden and McHenry awards from the Nutrition Society of Canada and the Conrad Elvehjem Award from the American Institute of Nutrition as well as recognition through the Atwater Memorial (U.S.) and Lord Boyd Orr (U.K.) lectureships. Dr. Beaton holds B.A., M.A., and Ph.D. degrees from the University of Toronto.

JAMES D. COOK is Phillips Professor of Medicine and Director, Division of Hematology, at the University of Kansas Medical Center, Kansas City. Dr. Cook is a member of the International Nutrition Anemia Consultative Group and an international consultant in hematology and anemias. He is a fellow of the American College of Physicians and member of the American Society for Hematology and the American Society for Clinical Nutrition. Dr. Cook holds M.D., C.M., and M.Sc. degrees from Queen's University, Kingston, Ontario, Canada.

PETER R. DALLMAN (consultant) recently retired as Professor of Pediatrics, School of Medicine, University of California at San Francisco. He is author of the background paper (Appendix B) developed for the present committee. Dr. Dallman's research is in the area of iron nutrition and iron metablolism. Dr. Dallman served on the Food and Nutrition Board's Subcommittee on Nutrition During Pregnancy and the Subcommittee on a Clinical Applications Guide of the Committee on Nutrition During Pregnancy and Lactation. He also has served on the Committee on Nutrition, American Academy of Pediatrics, and is a former chairman of the Nutrition Study Section at the National Institutes of Health, U.S. Department of Health and Human Services. Dr. Dallman holds a B.S. from Dartmouth College and an M.D. from Harvard Medical School.

SAMUEL J. FOMON is Professor Emeritus in the College of Medicine, University of Iowa. He is the author of numerous publications on infant nutrition and is a past chair of the Committee on Nutrition of the American Academy of Pediatrics. He has also served as president of the American Institute of Nutrition and the American Society for Clinical Nutrition and is an honorary member of the American Dietetic Association. In addition to honors from Western European and Latin American countries, Dr. Fomon has received the McCollum Award of the American Society for Clinical Nutrition, the U.S. Food and Drug Administration Commissioner's Special Citation, the Conrad A. Elvehjem Award of the American Institute of Nutrition, and the Bristol-Meyers Squibb/Mead Johnson Award for Distinguished Achievement in Nutrition Research. Dr. Fomon holds an A.B. from Harvard University and an M.D. from the University of Pennsylvania.

JANET L. MITCHELL is Chief of Perinatology, Department of Obstetrics and Gynecology at Harlem Hospital Center, New York, New York. Dr.

Mitchell was previously director of Ambulatory Perinatology at Beth Israel Hospital, Boston, Massachusetts, and served as an obstetrical consultant to the Bureau of Maternity Services and Family Planning for the New York City Department of Health. She is a member of the Governing Council, Maternal and Child Health Section, American Public Health Association; a fellow in the American College of Obstetricians and Gynecologists; and a member of the New England Medical Society, an affiliate of the National Medical Association. Dr. Mitchell holds an A.B. from Mount Holyoke College, an M.D. from Howard University, and an M.P.H. from the Harvard University School of Public Health.

DAVID RUSH is Head of the Epidemiology Program, U.S. Department of Agriculture's (USDA) Human Nutrition Research Center on Aging at Tufts University, and Professor of Nutrition, Community Health, and Pediatrics at Tufts University, Boston, Massachusetts. Dr. Rush previously held positions with the Albert Einstein College of Medicine, the Columbia University College of Physicians and Surgeons, and the University of Rochester and has served as an Epidemic Intelligence Service Officer with the U.S. Centers for Disease Control. Dr. Rush was a member of the Food and Nutrition Board's Subcommittee on Nutrition During Lactation of the Committee on Nutrition During Pregnancy and Lactation. He was principal investigator for the 1981–1986 national evaluation of the USDA Special Supplemental Food Program for Women, Infants, and Children. He is a member of the Society for Pediatric Research, the American Pediatric Society, the Perinatal Research Society, the American Institute of Nutrition, and the American Society of Clinical Nutrition; is a fellow of the American College of Epidemiology; and is past-president of the Society for Epidemiology in Research. Dr. Rush holds A.B. and M.D. degrees from Harvard University.

STAFF

CATHERINE E. WOTEKI is Director of the Institute of Medicine's (IOM) Food and Nutrition Board (FNB). Prior to joining the IOM, she was Deputy Director of the Division of Health Examination Statistics, National Center for Health Statistics, U.S. Department of Health and Human Services. She has served in important health posts at the Office of Technology Assessment of the U.S. Congress and at the U.S. Department of Agriculture's Human Nutrition Information Service. Dr. Woteki is coeditor of the FNB publication *Eat For Life: The Food and Nutrition Board's Guide to Reducing Your Risk of Chronic Disease*. She was a recipient of an IOM Distinguished Staff Award in 1991 and holds various honors from the Public Health Service, U.S. Department of Health and Human Services. Dr. Woteki currently serves as a member of the Council on Research of the American Dietetic Association and on the editorial advisory board of the American Institute of Nutrition. Dr. Woteki holds a B.S. from Mary Washington College, Fredricksburg, Virginia, and M.S. and Ph.D. degrees from Virginia Polytechnic Institute and State University, Blacksburg.

ROBERT EARL has been a Program Officer with the Food and Nutrition Board (FNB) since 1990. In addition to working with the Committee on the Prevention, Detection, and Management of Iron Deficiency Anemia Among U.S. Children and Women of Childbearing Age, he is Project Director of the FNB's Food Forum and was Staff Officer of studies by the Committee on the Nutrition Components of Food Labeling and the Committee on State Food Labeling. Prior to joining the Institute of Medicine, Mr. Earl was Administrator of Government Affairs for the American Dietetic Association in Washington, D.C. Previously, he was statewide nutrition consultant for adult health, chronic disease, and health promotion programs with the Texas Department of Health, Austin. Mr. Earl is currently President of the District of Columbia Metropolitan Area Dietetic Association and is a member of Delta Omega National Public Health Honorary Society. Mr. Earl holds a B.S. from the University of Michigan, Ann Arbor, an M.P.H. from the University of North Carolina at Chapel Hill, and is working on a doctorate in public policy at the Center for Public Administration and Policy at Virginia Polytechnic Institute and State University, Falls Church.

MARCIA S. LEWIS is the Administrative Assistant for the Food and Nutrition Board (FNB) and is Project Assistant for the Committee on the Prevention, Detection, and Management of Iron Deficiency Anemia Among U.S. Children and Women of Childbearing Age. Before becoming the Administrative Assistant to the FNB, Ms. Lewis was the Project Assistant for the Committee on Food Chemicals Codex and the Committee on Food Additives Survey. Before joining the Institute of Medicine, Ms. Lewis was a teacher, a technical writer, and an editor. She holds a B.A. degree and a Masters Certificate in editing and publishing from the George Washington University, Washington, D.C.

MICHAEL K. HAYES has been an editorial consultant with the National Academy of Sciences since 1985. He has edited numerous publications for the Institute of Medicine, including *Nutrition During Pregnancy and Lactation*, *Nutrition During Pregnancy and Lactation: An Implementation Guide*, *Nutrition Labeling*, *Adverse Effects of Pertussis and Rubella Vaccines*, *The Children's Vaccine Initiative: Achieving the Vision*, and *Adverse Events Associated with Childhood Vaccines*. Mr. Hayes also edits research articles published in *Antimicrobial Agents and Chemotherapy* and the *Journal of Clinical Microbiology*, both of which are publications of the American Society for Microbiology. He holds a B.A. from the University of Kansas, Lawrence.